SECRETS

OF THE

SEXUALLY

SATISFIED

WOMAN

Ten Keys

to Unlocking

Ultimate

Pleasure

SECRETS
OF THE
SEXUALLY
SATISFIED
WOMAN

Laura Berman, Ph.D., and Jennifer Berman, M.D.

with Alice Burdick Schweiger

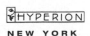

NEW YORK

PHOTO PERMISSIONS

p. 89 © Dawn Danby and Paul Waggoner
p. 114 © Dawn Danby
p. 182 © Dawn Danby and Paul Waggoner

ISBN 0-7868-6919-4

Book design by Richard Oriolo

Printed in the U.S.A.

This book is dedicated to

the sexually satisfied woman

inside each of you.

May you find her and

release her in all her glory!

Contents

Acknowledgments ix

Introduction 1

ONE Communication In and Out of the Bedroom: How Sexually Satisfied Women Get Their Message Across, and How You Can, Too 7

TWO Emotional Well-being: Feeling Self-confident, Stable, Secure, and Good About Yourself 25

THREE Relationship Health: *The* Emotional Connection 53

FOUR Self-stimulation 85

FIVE Arousal, Lubrication, and Orgasm 101

SIX Addressing Your Past 129

SEVEN Accepting and Overcoming Physical Obstacles 159

EIGHT Sexual Empowerment 189

NINE Attitudes and Sex Across the Generations 203

Final Thoughts 229

Appendix

Notes 231

Products 235

Suggested Reading 237

Resources 241

The Women's Sexual Satisfaction Survey 247

Acknowledgments

There are so many to thank—without them this book would not have been possible. First, thank you so much to Alice Burdick Schweiger, who worked so diligently to put our words and thoughts to paper and make them come alive. Also a special loving thanks to her mother, Jeannette Burdick, who passed away during the writing of this book. Thank you also to Binky Urban, our agent, who helped to carry us through this process and helped to make this book a reality. As always, we consider ourselves truly lucky to have you on our side! Special thanks to our publisher, Hyperion, and our editor, Gretchen Young.

The Women's Sexual Satisfaction Survey (WSSS) would not have been possible without the support of Lifetime television as well as an unrestricted educational grant from Procter and Gamble. We thank both companies for their investment in women's sexual health and their willingness to assist with moving this project forward. We also want to thank the Rand Corporation for their invaluable help in developing the WSSS, especially Sandra Berry and Chloe Bird. Thank you also to REDA International, the company that collected the data and pulled it all together, especially Joan Wang and Elham Aldredge. Also a big thank-you to Martin Lee, who has always made himself available and was instrumental in helping us start to make sense of the wealth of data we were able to collect. Laura Bogart, of RAND, provided the analyses we requested.

There are so many others who have supported us and made this book possible.

FROM LAURA

A huge thank-you to all of the staff at the Berman Center who provided the crucial logistical support as well as insights and perspectives that added so much to our interpretation of the findings: Jeremy Charles, Ann Marie Czerwinski, Ron Daniel, Becky Jeffers, Dee Hartmann, Darci Hemesath, Jane Lee, Bill McDunn, Kathy Monke, Jeanine Ramirez, Lynne Reich, Suzanne Roth, Nayia Sivulka, Michelle Wagenknecht, Martha Weinfurter, and April Wright.

Thank you to the folks at NEWSHE.com, Wendy Claunch, Stan Felder, Myron Murdock, and Mukesh Pitroda, and the staff at the *Dr. Laura Berman Show*, all of whom work so hard every day to get the message out there to women. I also want to thank my agent, Hayden Meyer from United Talent Agency, for his enthusiasm and guidance, and Greg Suess, Jay Froberg, and Bernie Cahill from Roar for their creativity and direction.

I have so much appreciation for my friends who have consistently lent me not only a shoulder and an ear but a dose of positive energy, even when they had little to spare. Most especially: Elizabeth Evans, Jennifer Gilbert, Marla Henderson, Niamh King, Marilyn Levitt, Saira Mohan, Elise Paschen, and Dana Weinstein. Thank you to my family: our parents, Linda and Irwin Berman; our grandmothers, Teal Friedman and Jean Berman; my sons, Ethan and Sammie; and most of all the biggest thank-you to my husband, Sam Chapman, who has been my supporter, champion, and muse. You kept me going even when I didn't think I could make it, and have helped me realize my greatest dreams. The journey is just beginning.

FROM JENNIFER

I want to thank my friends, family, and office staff who put up with me through this long journey. I am particularly grateful to my husband, Greg, for his contribution to the format, content, and statistical analyses. I love you and thank you for making me a satisfied woman!

SECRETS

OF THE

SEXUALLY

SATISFIED

WOMAN

Introduction

One of the greatest mysteries of life is what constitutes a woman's sexual satisfaction. This book is about solving that mystery. It's about making sexual Nirvana an achievable goal, and unlocking the secrets to extraordinary lovemaking.

It's safe to say that many of us strive to reach the pinnacle of sexual bliss. It's why we read the magazine articles, buy the books, and watch television with such a fervent interest when there is something in the news about ecstasy in the bedroom. Sex is a central part of who we are—it's a part of the fabric of our relationships and our society. Most women agree that sex is much more than our genitals, and at the same time, it is not just a state of mind.

There is a complex relationship between life circumstances, health factors, and our sexuality, often barely understood even by experts in the field. We are sisters and doctors—Laura a therapist, Jennifer a physician. Our careers are focused on helping women find sexual pleasure. For years, women have been talking to us about their sensual aspirations, regardless of their age, marital status, race, and religion.

We have built two of the premier centers for research and treatment of female sexuality: Laura is clinical assistant professor of OB/GYN and psychiatry at Northwestern Memorial Hospital in Chicago and directs the Berman Center there, and Jennifer is assistant professor of urology at the David Geffen School of Medicine at UCLA in Los Angeles and directs the Female Sexual Medical Center there. The combination of our backgrounds led us to take a multifaceted, mind-body approach to working with the total woman.

We find there has been a lack of understanding between therapists and the medical establishment that has led to a piecemeal treatment approach to women's sexuality. There is a common frustration among our female patients, as so much focus in the medical community is on male sexuality, male sexual function, and getting an erection long enough to have intercourse. This treatment gap derives from a lack of medical attention paid to women. Much of the focus has been on the clinical treatment of erectile dysfunction. This is in part a result of men pushing for an end point, namely an erection sufficient enough to perform.

While males often associate ultimate sexual pleasure with orgasm, for women it's much broader. It's an overall feeling a woman has about her love life. The FDA guidelines for new drugs are focused on orgasm as the main outcome variable to prove effectiveness, but it's not necessarily the most important factor.

Two years ago we began a journey to understand the complexity of women's sexual satisfaction. Rather than focus on negative aspects, we decided to take another approach. The better question, we thought, is to ask what are the secrets of people who celebrate their sex life and what can we learn from them? What components of their romantic lives lead to ecstasy under the sheets? Drawing from our personal experience with the thousands of women we've treated, as well as our peers and published literature, we created a study that measured sexual satisfaction.

We asked a wide range of questions relating to lifestyle, mental and physical health, and sexual attitudes and behavior. The questions were designed as a validated measure of sexual satisfaction. By comparing the results we were able to determine how the various life factors correlated. In essence, we wanted to find the top ten keys to help every woman unlock the sexually satisfied woman inside.

THE WOMEN'S SEXUAL SATISFACTION SURVEY (WSSS)

Our goal was to carry out this study in the most scientific way possible. We selected a nationwide sample of women by random-digit telephone calling. A total of 2,604 women, eighteen and over, participated in the survey, and of them, 41 percent felt that having a satisfying sex life is very important, a pleasantly surprising number. There was no notable difference in sexual satisfaction as far as income, employment, education, or race. In the overall sample, 49 percent had a high school diploma or less, and 51 percent had some vocational school, college, or more.

The respondents ranged in age from eighteen to seventy-one. The breakdown by age group is:

18–24 years, 14 percent
25–34 years, 21 percent
35–44 years, 24 percent
45–54 years, 20 percent
55–64 years, 13 percent
65–71 years, 8 percent

The women were of varied ethnic backgrounds, although predominately white: 66 percent Caucasian, 12 percent African American, 11 percent Hispanic, 3 percent Asian/Pacific, 3 percent mixed race, 3 percent Native American, and 3 percent other. (This adds up to 101 percent due to rounding off the numbers.) All of the women resided in the contiguous United States.

In analyzing the survey results for this book, we assessed what these women have in common, such as their state of mind, their outlook on life, their sexual function, and the nature of their relationships. (See the Appendix for survey questions.)

OUR GOAL

In writing this book we hope to help all women reach their ultimate passionate connection. We want them to look forward to and cherish their sex lives, which contributes greatly to general health and wellness. In fact, studies have shown that sexual satisfaction is an important factor in marital happiness, and sexual dissatisfaction is associated with divorce.

We hope to inform and empower women, encourage them to take control of their sexuality, and overcome hurdles. We want women to feel comfortable advocating for their sexual needs and know they have the tools necessary to accomplish it. We also want to dispel some of the myths.

In our first book, *For Women Only: A Revolutionary Guide to Reclaiming Your Sex Life,* we armed women with information about their bodies and sexual response, and offered treatment options when they are faced with sexual dysfunction. We focused on physical difficulties and sexual stumbling blocks. The premise was that all women should feel entitled to their sexuality, and we want to build on that idea. This is the first national study that compares multiple life factors to measures of sexual satisfaction. From the findings, we are able to offer advice on maximizing sexual function.

Based on our clinical experience, along with the survey results, the following are ten key components to sexual satisfaction:

1. **Sexual communication in and out of the bedroom**
2. **Relationship health—emotional and physical connectedness**
3. **Strong emotional health and social support**

4. **Self-stimulation**

5. **Addressing your past**

6. **Orgasm**

7. **Arousal**

8. **Lubrication**

9. **Accepting and overcoming physical obstacles**

10. **Sexual empowerment**

In this book we will explore these components. We have devised quizzes, tips, rules, and guidelines. In the process of trying to attain sexual satisfaction, there will be inevitable struggles and soul-searching. You may revisit your past and reevaluate your relationships and expectations. You may have to change the way you think about sex, yourself, and your partner. It may mean changing your attitudes, confronting your weaknesses, and assessing your emotional well-being with an open mind. You may find our advice easy to follow, or you may find it just the first step on your journey to sexual health. It is important to note that deep-rooted problems can be hard to fix, and when solutions are too challenging, therapy may be indicated. (See the Appendix on how to choose a therapist and type of treatment.)

This book is for every woman. Those who are sexually satisfied will want to continue to enhance their romantic lives, and those who are not will want to find ways for improvement.

ONE

Communication In and Out of the Bedroom

How Sexually Satisfied Women Get Their Message Across, and How You Can, Too

t's clear from our findings that being able to communicate your needs is a key to great sex. Sexually satisfied women are comfortable telling their partners what they want. Married or not, they know the importance of expressing their feelings and getting the most out of lovemaking.

FINDINGS FROM THE WOMEN'S SEXUAL SATISFACTION SURVEY

Sexual communication is a verbal and nonverbal dialogue about sex. The women who are sexually satisfied reported:

- They communicate with their partner openly about sex.
- They feel emotionally and physically connected/intimate with their partner.
- They believe both men and women enjoy sex equally.

Comparisons between married women and singles in sexual communication showed:

- Married and single women have similar sexual communication styles.
- Married, single, and never-married women use both nonverbal and verbal communication techniques to let their partners know what they like in bed.
- Married women were significantly more likely than unmarried women to have good communication with their partner about sex.

Kristen's Story

Kristen, age thirty-four, had been sexual with her husband, Bo, also thirty-four, for three years by the time they were married. But even after two years of marriage, she mostly reached orgasm through self-stimulation, rarely with her husband. She attributed this to his technique and just accepted his ho-hum lovemaking. As one might imagine, over time she became increasingly less satisfied, as well as unmotivated to have sex at all. Kristen began to believe the reason she reached orgasm alone and not with her husband was because they were out of sync. He did not know how or where to stimulate her, or how to apply the right pressure to her clitoris.

The idea of admitting to him that he couldn't satisfy her was daunting. She thought long and hard and finally mustered up the courage, broached the subject, and talked about what aroused her sexually. She started by letting his hand rest on hers while she self-stimulated, which was a huge feat because she found it very embarrassing. It didn't take long before he learned to mirror what she was doing. They continued an ongoing dialogue and she was able to reach orgasm with him.

> **Women who used both words and guiding in communicating their sexual desires to their partner were more sexually satisfied than those who used touching only.**

There is no doubt that expressing your desires can make you feel vulnerable and uncomfortable. Yet sexual satisfaction isn't about guesswork or assumptions, it's about telling your partner what pleases you and eliminating barriers. You can't improve your sexual intimacy without sharing and making your preferences, dislikes, pleasures, and fantasies known.

If you struggle with sexual communication and feel that you want to tune up your skills, there are several rules of thumb that sexually satisfied women follow to communicate their deepest, darkest wants and needs:

Speak up.
What to do: Bring up the subject gently and offer reassurance. Slant things on a more upbeat note. Say: "I love what you are doing, keep doing it that way," or "That feels great." Avoid the downer approach, saying things like: "It bothers me when you touch me there."

Be positive.

What to do: Make sure the positive feedback outweighs the negative. If your partner feels effective, he (or she) will be more open to further suggestions and less likely to shut down.

Take a risk.

What to do: Try more physical stimulation and foreplay or act out a fantasy. Don't be afraid to speak your mind. Without being vocal about your desires it's difficult to achieve sexual satisfaction. Sometimes it's scary to reveal your inner secrets, but be brave, it will pay off.

Lead the way.

What to do: Take your hand and touch yourself the way you want, or let your partner put his hand on yours while you guide the way. Men want to be our sexual white knights, they just don't know how. Even if they have been intimate with numerous women, unless they are with someone who knows her body and is able to communicate with them, they can be clueless. It's up to the woman to understand her body and direct her partner in and out of the bedroom.

Keep an open mind.

What to do: Be flexible. Your partner probably has ideas of what's exciting, so it's important to hear what he has to say. Communication works both ways. Don't be defensive when you get a taste of your own medicine.

Be patient.

What to do: Be encouraging and understand that it may take time to feel less awkward or to have your requests effectively implemented. It may take several tries before your partner gets it right.

Don't pull out the measuring stick.

What to do: Concentrate on the present relationship. If you had another partner who sent shivers down your spine, don't bring it up. Nothing pours cold water on a good sex life like being compared to a past lover, especially if the comparison is not favorable!

Live in the present tense.

What to do: Stick to the here and now. What's done is done. Dredging up past arguments or difficulties in your relationship will only alienate your partner.

Avoid being judgmental.

What to do: Take your partner's feelings into consideration. Do not express your needs with any anger or contempt. And definitely avoid insults about him or his anatomy!

If you have a sensitive issue you want to bring into the open, it's better to talk about it outside of the bedroom. Stay away from discussing problems in the midst of sexual activity because it's easy to feel very vulnerable in the middle of sex. It's a surefire mood spoiler.

TEST THE WATERS: TIPS FOR BREAKING THE ICE

Expressing your sexual desires doesn't always come easy. In fact, many women are painfully shy when it comes to exposing their deepest wishes. For some, it's the fear of being rejected, for others it's the concern of being too kinky for their partner's tastes. If you are too bashful to bring up what arouses you, try some of these techniques.

Start off slow.

What to do: Begin with a simple request that is easily accomplished. Maybe it's to spend more time on foreplay or a certain body part you want to have kissed. This way it's not threatening and will not only make you more comfortable, but will set the stage for further pleasures.

Use words of affection.

What to do: Begin by calling your partner a pet or endearing name, like honey or sweetheart—as corny as that may sound. Start with something like: "Sweetheart, I love when you rub my——. Can you do that more often?"

Put it in writing.

What to do: Send your sexy idea in a note or e-mail. This can be helpful if there is something new you want to try in the bedroom and are afraid to say out loud. Jotting it down on paper may be less intimidating.

Have fun.

What to do: Turn communicating into an exploratory game. Say: "I will show you how and where I want to be kissed if you show me."

SEXY TALK: WAYS FOR HEATING UP THE MOMENT

Once you have broken the ice, think about heating up the moment with erotic talk—in other words, speaking to your partner in graphic sexual language. It's the sexually satisfied woman's way to express passion, heighten the arousal process, and add a sensual dimension to lovemaking. Talking dirty doesn't come naturally, but it's a way to enhance the sexual encounter through the sense of hearing. Sure, it means taking a risk, but it can be a bonding experience.

No one ever teaches us how to be sexy, talk raunchy, or exhibit our lusty side. We are not all born with the capability to be seductive. How do we learn to talk sexy to the one we love? How do we know we are effective when we attempt to be lustful? Some women have the gift of an active imagination and the ability to be a great storyteller and sensual talker. Others find inspiration from steamy love novels and instructional books. If you are tongue-tied and at a loss for where to begin, consider these tried-and-true secrets of seduction.

Take your time.

What to do: Begin with a conversation about what feels good sexually and gradually lead into more graphic language. Start off with *I*'s. For example, fill in the blanks: "I would like for you to ____." "I feel so ____ when you ____ me." "I want to ____ your ____." "I love to look at your ____."

Step it up and strut your stuff.

What to do: If the first step went well, move into steamier conversation. Try completing the following sentences: "____ me now!" "____ my ____." "I want to feel your ____ against my ____." "I want you to touch my ____." "My ____ loves the way your ____ feels."

Practice makes perfect.

What to do: Before you say these things to your partner, practice saying them aloud, alone, in front of the mirror. The goal is to look and sound as natural as possible. You may feel silly at first, but practice makes perfect.

To do it, you gotta know it.
What to do: Pick up a sexually explicit book and read it to yourself, then read it aloud to your partner—it can be a fun activity or serve as foreplay. *The Story of O* by Pauline Reage is a great book to consider.

Be creative.
What to do: Describe an erotic scenario and leave it in a note where your partner can find it.

Make a list of sexy words and phrases.
What to do: Think of what to say before, during, and after sex. Keep it in a safe, private place. It is likely, once you have written the words down, that you won't forget them.

Cuddle up and whisper in his ear.
What to do: Snuggle in the arms of your partner, get him in the mood for whatever explicit conversation you may introduce.

Make a call.
What to do: Go into another room and phone him from your cell. In detail, tell him what you'd like to try.

Watch an X-rated video for inspiration.
What to do: Rent the movie on cable TV or at the nearest video store. It can bring up ideas not only of what to say, but how to say it. It's okay to plagiarize!

STARTING YOUR ENGINE

Don't forget to warm up! The preliminary activities that lead to a sexual encounter are a key part of sexual communication, and often set the overall tone. Sometimes they are extremely passionate and intense, sometimes softer and sweeter.

For starters, ambience is everything. Burning candles, massage oils, and incense all enhance the sexual experience. In creating a seductive environment, soft music, low lights, and sweet smells communicate a desire to be sexual with your partner. An enticing setting may be more powerful and telling than words.

Pay attention to comfort—creature comforts are everything. Changing the sheets to a higher thread count, or perhaps to satin or silk, is conducive to spicy sex and makes you feel more sensual.

If you have a romantic evening planned, signal ahead with an e-mail or a phone call during the day about your sexual intentions. The anticipation will build, making the sexual encounter more exciting. Or better yet, leave a risqué note about a new position you want to try. It's bound to ignite the flames of passion.

Check out these sexy signals that sexually satisfied women use for setting the sensual stage and "communicating" they are ready for love:

Remember, it's all in the delivery.

What to do: Speak in a sexy, low tone. Even a soft whisper directly in your partner's ear can be an aphrodisiac. Because your face will be hidden, it might be a little less embarrassing. Your partner will enjoy the content of what you are saying, as well as the sensation of your breath in his ear, which is a key erogenous zone.

Reminisce and relish past sexual adventures together.

What to do: Snuggle up on the couch and recall mind-blowing sexual encounters that you had with your partner. This will definitely lead to some steamy moments.

Surprise, surprise.

What to do: When your partner is in the shower, pop in and offer to wash him from head to toe. Maybe make an unexpected visit to work with lunch in tow, or show up naked while he's doing chores or working at home. The element of surprise will put a smile on his face and set the mood.

A few words go a long way.

What to do: Leave him little love notes in his pockets, briefcase, or underwear drawer. Or mark your lovemaking intentions with lipstick on the mirror.

Plan a romantic escape.

What to do: Book a hotel room for the night. Surprising your partner with a key to a hotel room will guarantee a sizzling evening. Tell the front desk you do not want to be disturbed. Or just plan a special afternoon or evening outing—it doesn't need to be an overnight.

IT'S NOT ALL IN WHAT YOU SAY, BUT WHAT YOU DO

Although words are usually the best way to communicate, if you are uneasy being verbally direct, and find it too intimidating, then consider nonverbal cues. You can get your message across without uttering a single word. Nonverbal cues can be used both when you want to be sexual, and in the heat of the moment.

Let's say you are ready to embark on a sexual encounter but are reluctant to be the initiator, and you would rather reach out without speaking. No problem. The following are some ways sexually satisfied women let their partners know through body language that they are ready for love:

Make eye contact.
What to do: Whether dining with friends or noisy kids, catch your partner's eye at the dinner table. A loving gaze can convey your thoughts through your eyes and be very arousing. The long stare can be very exciting for the recipient, and the intentions can be clear.

Give an affectionate stroke or touch.
What to do: A prolonged hug, a rub on the arm, or a long neck or back massage will get the message across much more effectively than a quick pat.

Sit up close and snuggle.
What to do: Shift your body so he can feel your body heat. Move closer to him on the couch. It's a clear invitation to the bedroom.

WHAT'S GOOD FOR THE GOOSE ISN'T ALWAYS GOOD FOR THE GANDER

Women and men are programmed very differently, especially when it comes to sexual stimulation. For a man, the pleasures of physical intimacy start with genital stimulation. They like to go straight to their partner's vulva and breasts, and in turn, have their penis stroked right away. Women, on the other hand, like to warm things up with rubbing and fondling before their genitals are actually touched. Many women are under the false belief that if their partner engages in little foreplay, or reaches orgasm quickly, they are not interested in pleasing them. In truth, men do want to satisfy and are usually more than willing to work up to intercourse. Although women are more apt to convey their feelings and men are more inclined to pull back, neither gender has an easy time communicating about sex. But mutual pleasure is possible. Consider these ways to enhance your sexual satisfaction during lovemaking:

Keep the water boiling: Foreplay is good.
What to do: Prolong the passion with foreplay. It makes the sexual experience more intense. Foreplay is not just genital stimulation, it's kissing, massaging, touching, fondling, and caressing, and it makes your orgasm more powerful. Prolonging the passion may require verbal communication, and it's okay to say you want more.

Focus on giving as well as receiving pleasure.
What to do: Be aware of your partner's reaction to your moves. Don't be afraid to ask your partner what he (or she) likes.

Don't give up too soon, but know when the party's over.
What to do: Remember that orgasm does not need to happen during sex. If your partner ejaculates too soon or you still want more, before, during, or after he reaches orgasm, have him focus on your sexual buildup and pleasure. If you are not in the mood or having a very difficult time reaching orgasm, it's okay to want to stop and cuddle. Don't feel guilty or bad about letting your partner know your feelings.

It's all right to say no, but it's all in the delivery. And keep in mind, he, and/or you, may get a second wind.

Spice it up with variety.

What to do: Sometimes have sex in your partner's favorite position, sometimes in yours. What about trying a new position? How about sex in a place other than bed? The back porch, perhaps? And break out the toys if you need to.

KEEP TALKING: FEEDBACK IS GOOD

Feedback he gets from your words, voice, and moans is the key to keeping the flames ignited and ensuring a repeat performance. For some couples, just talking about sex makes them aroused. Communicating your desires isn't only about enlightening your partner on how to stimulate you. It's also about creating a mood, sharing your fantasies, and reaffirming your sexual relationship. Here are two rules of thumb:

Show and tell.

What to do: Be a good sexual communicator. Be knowledgeable about your body—you are the expert. Sexually satisfied women know what type of stimulation they like and what they need to achieve orgasm. In the midst of being aroused, a moan, a sigh, a simple "yes" will also give the message to keep on going. Or, how about establishing a cue of reassurance? A smile, a wink, or a nod should work. There is nothing wrong with gestures—sometimes they speak loud and clear.

Take ownership.

What to do: Be in charge. In order to be satisfied, you need to take ownership of your sexuality and not rely on your partner. Sexually satisfied women do not rely on their partner to sexually satisfy them, or believe it's their partner's responsibility to deliver them into the throes of ecstasy.

THE AFTERGLOW

Instead of dozing off after sex, think about basking in postcoital passion. That's what many sexually satisfied women enjoy. While emotions are still high, they exchange thoughts. Something light will do, it doesn't have to be intensely deep. The delicate period after sex can be a time to bond, to maintain a level of comfort. Just holding each other, watching a movie, cuddling quietly, munching on snacks are all connecting experiences. Just being with each other after something so intimate enhances the union.

To prolong the intimacy and keep your partner in place before the mood changes, incorporate some TLC, or something he may enjoy. Give him a back rub, bring him something to eat, pop in a video, and he will be more willing to stick around. Don't turn on the TV and start flipping through channels. Don't get up to check your e-mail—keep the computer off. Think of it as sacred space and time. If you find your partner isn't responding to your attempts, and he wants to jump out of bed, talk to him about it. If the afterglow lasts long enough, you may be able to reinspire another sexual encounter.

MARRIED OR SINGLE, BETTER SAFE THAN SORRY

Communicating means speaking up for your safety. It means being your own advocate. So if you are worried about pulling out a condom or setting ground rules, don't be. Partaking in a safe-sex discussion and using protection should be a given. If your partner doesn't initiate the conversation, be assertive and bring it up yourself. This should be a priority, considering the risk of HIV and STDs, as well as getting pregnant. If a potential sexual partner resists, take a strong stance. Don't give in. This should not be negotiable for anyone—sexually satisfied women, or anyone struggling to better their sex lives.

Sometimes you need to bargain for safer sex. It may require taking responsibility for the condom and carrying it with you. You can even make it a part of foreplay by applying the condom in an erotic fashion—with your mouth, for example. If your partner resists using protection, claiming he doesn't have a disease and that sex doesn't feel as good with a prophylactic, don't compromise. Women are increasingly becoming infected with HIV, and having unprotected sex isn't worth the danger.

Teenagers and young adults in particular may be intimidated to initiate the discussion, but safe-sex practices are essential. The dialogue should be ongoing and a key component in building and maintaining a trusting relationship. It should be stressed that it's for mutual protection, not just yours. Abstinence would be a better choice than indulging in unprotected sex.

In monogamous relationships where both parties use condoms and/or have been tested and they know the only risk they face is pregnancy, there is less concern and anxiety, which lends itself to greater sexual response and sexual satisfaction. Couples in a monogamous relationship also have the advantage of not having to worry about the danger of disease.

SEXUAL COMMUNICATION TEST

Wondering how you fare in the sexual communication arena? Take this test and see if you need to hone your skills—answer yes or no.

- Do you let your partner know when you are ready for sex?
- How would your partner answer that question—does he always know when you want to have sex?
- Do you verbally and nonverbally communicate your sexual needs?
- Does your partner verbally and nonverbally communicate his sexual needs?
- Do you express your pleasure through words and actions?
- Do you let your partner know when he/she sexually pleases you?
- Do you feel comfortable sharing your disappointment when you are dissatisfied with your sex life?
- Do you share your sexual fantasies with your partner?
- Do you feel competent in your sexual communication ability?

SCORING

If you answered "yes" to:

0–3 OUT OF THE 9 ITEMS: You need to improve your communicating skills. You may want to consider some of our tips. It's clear you need to do some work and understand it's a key part of your sexual health.

4–6 OUT OF THE 9 ITEMS: You have some strengths but are not completely comfortable communicating. Your skills aren't bad, but there is room for improvement.

7–9 OUT OF THE 9 ITEMS: You are a pretty good communicator. If you scored on the lower end, there is still some room for improvement. If you scored on the higher end, you are in good shape.

BOTTOM LINE FOR SEXUAL COMMUNICATION, MARRIED OR SINGLE

If you establish a pattern of communicating effectively outside of the bedroom, it will be easier for you to be expressive about issues that occur in the bedroom. Women who have a good support system in their partner and can easily share their thoughts, fears, insecurities, emotions, and challenges are more apt to feel an emotional intimacy and connection. Sound too good to be true? It's not, but it does take work and it isn't easy. Sexually satisfied women communicate. They are secure and comfortable using verbal, nonverbal, and visual cues with their partners.

While our survey found married women communicated better overall, it shouldn't be assumed that just because a woman is married she is automatically a good sexual communicator. We have seen many married women who are uncomfortable talking about their sexual needs to their husbands. Depending on the nature of the relationship, you can be married and feel insecure, or be divorced or single and feel secure. If you are in a committed relationship where you feel safe and not judged by your partner, and are able to take responsibility for your arousal, you are much more likely to feel comfortable revealing what turns you on, married or not.

Of those currently married/cohabitating, or with a partner,

    10 percent use words

    5 percent use touch/guiding

    85 percent use both

All part of the bottom line, when you are in a relationship for a long time, it's easier to communicate because you understand each other and there is a certain established comfort level. Communication takes time, requires trust, and cannot be unilateral. However, while couples in long-term relationships may have an advantage, since they know each other so well, the novelty eventually wears off and they have to work hard to keep the flames ignited.

While married women reported having better sexual communication than unmarried women, there was no difference in their ability to communicate, or in their style. These findings suggest that regardless of marital status, women tend to behave similarly.

> 70 percent of married/cohabiting, 65 percent formerly married/cohabiting, 71 percent never-married women reported that they tell their partner what to or what not to do sexually, most or all of the time.

Footnote from the Doctors Berman

There may be factors that impede a woman's ability or desire to communicate sexually with her partner, such as sexual dysfunction, mental or physical health problems, history of abuse or trauma, significant relationship difficulties, life stresses relating to children or finances, and self-esteem issues. If you are completely disinterested or unable to communicate with your partner, you should consider discussing this with your health care provider, as there may be physical or emotional factors that need to be addressed and attended to.

Emotional Well-being

Feeling Self-confident, Stable, Secure, and Good About Yourself

We found that for the sexually satisfied woman, a healthy sex life goes hand in hand with a healthy emotional life. In our survey, the women who said they enjoyed life were also more content with their sex life. This is hardly surprising, since it's difficult to have a satisfying sexual relationship when you are unhappy, anxious, or stressed. We are not the only ones to come to this conclusion.

FINDINGS FROM THE WOMEN'S SEXUAL SATISFACTION SURVEY

Compared to women who are not sexually satisfied, women who are reported:

- They enjoy life and have healthy sex lives.
- They say they feel happy most of the time.
- They place importance on sexual satisfaction.
- They perceive themselves as physically attractive.

A poll of 3,100 people ages eighteen to fifty-nine at the National Opinion Research Center at the University of Chicago found a high correlation between frequency of sex and level of happiness.

Overcoming Stress:
Melanie's Story

Melanie was in her late forties when her aging parents became very ill, and as their only daughter, she was responsible for their health needs. Taking care of her parents was nothing new to her. Growing up, Melanie's mother and father suffered from depression and they took their hardships out on her. She spent a lifetime tending to her parents' emotional needs and now she was tending to their physical needs as well. Even if Melanie wasn't home with her parents, they were calling her on the phone, which was a never-ending burden. To make matters worse, her parents were not only ungrateful, they were critical and taxing.

No matter how much she tried to be there for her parents, Melanie constantly felt guilty and found it impossible to build a life of her own. Divorced and living with her teenage daughter, she had no support system. Not only did Melanie have poor self-esteem, she never had a healthy, satisfying sex life, much less a happy life in general. When she did have sex, she felt self-conscious and unsatisfied. Our goal was to work with her to improve her self-esteem as well as her sexual life and happiness. She wanted to enjoy sex without feeling helpless and hopeless, and without a heavy cloud hanging over her head.

Melanie's first line of action was to try to overcome stress. She developed skills to relax, learned how to take deep breaths when she found her heart racing, and started using yoga as a means of relaxation. In the evening, especially, she found yoga most effective. Her next step was to set up boundaries with her parents. She started off setting up small boundaries. She didn't call them back immediately after they phoned her; instead, she waited until it was convenient. She learned to stand up for herself, and say no to anything that would be hurtful to her. At first her parents resisted, but eventually they accepted Melanie's newfound independence. Through therapy she was able to see that her parents' issues were really about them and not her, and she finally felt she was in control of her life. She gained confidence that transferred over to her sex life. She began to venture out, was less anxious, socialized more, and started to explore her sexuality.

All of us know women like Melanie. Everyone experiences some stress in life. It's even expected in today's world, whether it's taking care of elderly parents, as with Melanie, or taking care of the kids and/or working full-time. Many women experience much more stress than men, because they take on most of the child-rearing responsibilities, whether they have a job outside the home or not. The *Gallup Poll Monthly* reported 49 percent of women say they frequently experience stress compared to 34 percent of men.

It's a myth that stay-at-home moms live the life of leisure. They have PTA and school board meetings, carpooling, organizing the kids' activities and helping them with their homework, cooking and cleaning house, etcetera. As women, we tend to overtax ourselves and put everyone else first.

The stress that women face can undermine their ability to enjoy sex, let alone get in the mood. When there is a lack of sexual desire, it puts a strain on their relationships, creating guilt and even more stress.

Chronic stress can actually have physical effects on the body's immune system and lead to other illnesses. A study by Sheldon Cohen, Ph.D., at Carnegie Mellon University, found that people with high stress levels are more likely to develop colds or the flu than people with lower levels.

Stress can also trigger a hormonal chain reaction. Men typically fall into the "fight or flight" mode. When there is a threatening situation, the adrenaline in their body increases and travels to the cardiac and skeletal muscles to prepare for a "fight or flight" response. In addition to "fight or flight," women can also fall into the "tend and befriend" mode, where their oxytocin levels rise and they want to cuddle, be with their families, and nest. The theory is that when oxytocin levels go up, a protein called sex hormone–binding globulin (SHBG) also increases. SHBG is a protein in the body that binds testosterone to the cells. When SHBG is bound to testosterone, it is then not available to bind to the target tissue; so in effect, it is unavailable for the body to use for things like libido. That's why women who are under chronic stress will have lower libido, because their free testosterone levels are down.

Sure, sexually satisfied women experience stress, but they have and use the tools to keep it from interfering with their sex life. Although there are no quick fixes, here are tips we learned from sexually satisfied women that may help you get relief from stresses and worries in your life:

Make time for sex.
What to do: Carve out more time for fun in the bedroom—it's a great stress-buster. It's energizing and relaxing, and can get your mind

off your worries. The feel-good chemicals you get with orgasm can alleviate stress.

Pump up the volume.

What to do: Work out, walk, or participate in sports on a regular basis. It is a stress reliever, allows time to wind down, and increases endorphin levels, which are feel-good chemicals. It makes the body stronger, in better condition, and more easily able to sleep. We often recommend yoga. It's relaxing and good for the body as it's all about balance, stretching, and strength. Yoga requires concentration of positions, which helps to focus inward.

Lighten the load.

What to do: Identify what in your life is causing you extra tension. When you pinpoint the source, think of resolutions. For example, if you rush home from work to be with the kids, consider stopping for a cup of coffee, for some down time without pressure, even if it's just for a half hour.

Get your priorities straight.

What to do: Decide what's important in life. Assess a potential stressful situation. Before anxiety gets out of hand, ask yourself if it will really make a difference in your life in five years, or even five hours?

Pass the buck.

What to do: Don't be afraid to delegate. And remember, you can say no. It's okay to back off from commitments, and let go of the idea that if someone else does it, it won't be done as well.

Forget about perfection.

What to do: Understand that nobody's perfect and try being more laid back. Everything doesn't have to be flawless. It's okay to go to the grocery store to buy the cookies instead of baking them for the class bake sale. It's fine if the dishes aren't always washed.

Don't forget about yourself.

What to do: Attend to your needs by setting aside time for yourself. There is nothing selfish about going to the gym or getting a manicure or pedicure. Relationships will suffer and patience will be short without any R&R (rest and relaxation).

Get organized.

What to do: Write a "to do" list. Tackle one task at a time. This keeps you from being overextended. If something isn't an emergency, it can be put off for a day or two. Accept the fact that the list may never be completed. You may even consider hiring a part-time assistant, similar to a mother's helper, whether you are a stay-at-home mom or not. This may sound out of the realm of possibilities, but college and/or high school students may be looking for a way to make extra money and their fee may fit into your budget.

Bringing Lust Back into Your Life:
Beth's Story

Beth and her husband, Alec, professionals in their late thirties, were married for ten years. Week after week, day after day, their life followed the same routine: at the office from morning till night, a late dinner, a little television, and then off to bed. They felt they were in a rut and their sex life mimicked the rest of their life—dull and predictable. They weren't having sex as often, partly because they were tired and partly because they were bored. Beth and Alec entered into therapy with Laura in the hopes of finding a way to spice up their life. They tried new positions and explored each other's fantasies, but what seemed to be most helpful was embarking on an outdoor adventure together. At Laura's suggestion, they booked a white-water rafting weekend trip. Not only did they find the experience thrilling and daring, after it was over they were excited to go to a secluded area in the woods to have sex. Although this trip wasn't the key element that saved their marriage, they continued to challenge and enjoy themselves by sharing exciting adventures.

> **47 percent of the women surveyed found life exciting.**

Here are some of our suggestions for breaking out of an unhappy cycle or preventing yourself from spiraling into one:

Don't just get busy, do things you enjoy.

What to do: While a routine schedule feels safe and predictable, it can sap your energy level and ability to have fun. To combat this boredom trap, try to find ways to incorporate something new into your life, whether it's taking a dance or art class, joining a theater group, or learning karate. Even just a little change in your routine can jump-start other parts of your life—and your relationship. Broaden your horizons. If you have never studied art, take a class at the closest museum. Try out a sexual fantasy. Yes, change is hard and can feel scary at first, but pushing the envelope can give your life a jolt.

Tend to the fire.

What to do: Keep romance alive. Find quiet, romantic activities to do alone with your partner, like a walk in the park or a picnic. Consider creating a tradition of sitting outside every night for a short while with a glass of wine, after the kids are asleep, to share the day's events.

Climb every mountain.

What to do: Don't be afraid of adventure. Welcome it and look for challenging things to do together like hiking, mountain climbing, white-water rafting, mountain biking, etcetera. You'll be sure to get the adrenaline rush, which is bound to increase your sexual appetite. Excitement goes hand in hand with sexual energy. Couples don't have to climb Mount Everest to reap the benefits—even going to the gym or participating in a sport together can be energizing.

Try to get caught.

What to do: There's nothing like thrill sex, where getting caught is a possibility. Whether it's the backyard or a deserted corner of a beach or park, making love in an open or public space adds an element of danger and excitement.

Leave Yourself a Little Time for R&R: Jackie's Story

Jackie and her husband, Brian, wanted to get away but couldn't miss work. They also felt guilty about leaving their kids, since their time with them was limited. In therapy Laura suggested that they work out a system where every few months they would go to a local hotel for a night or two. Jackie loved this advice because she didn't have to worry about traveling and liked being close by and reachable in case of an emergency. With this arrangement, Jackie and Brian were able to sleep in, have time to engage in more relaxed sex, and enjoy a part of their city they couldn't when they were with their kids. It helped them reconnect as a couple. They had been caught up in the daily grind of life and most of their communication revolved around the household, work issues, and managing the family.

Going on a vacation with your partner, or even alone, will make a huge difference. We had another patient who would go on a silent retreat, where for forty-eight hours she didn't speak. The level of introspection that she found, the recharging of her emotional batteries and reorienting herself to her own spirituality, was revitalizing. When she returned, her relationship and sex life with her husband were met with a new energy. Getting away by yourself and reconnecting to who you are as a person, beyond a mother or a wife, is very important. Equally as important, if not more so, is getting away as a couple.

LOVE THYSELF

Feel good about yourself? How about a sense of self-worth—do you think you have it? Are you confident when you walk out the door? If you answered yes to all of these, chances are you have good self-esteem. It's the foundation for personal happiness and most people strive for it. The sexually satisfied woman certainly has it! Self-esteem is the evaluation of one's self, and a combination of self-confidence and self-respect. Jerry Minchinton, author of *Maximum Self-Esteem*, says, "How we feel about ourselves affects everything we do, say and think."

What's more, feeling good about ourselves and believing others perceive us positively can affect our sex life. We found that sexually satisfied women feel good about themselves. They experience themselves as worthwhile and deserving human beings. While we are all born with the capacity to have faith in ourselves, many of us struggle with self-doubt some, if not all, of the time. Self-esteem has to come from within. Everyone has self-esteem; it's a matter of whether it's good or poor.

How do you rank on the self-esteem scale? Take this simple quiz and see how you fare (answer yes or no):

- Are you an optimist?
- Do you expect good outcomes rather than the worst-case scenario?
- Do you feel worthy of other people's love and affection?
- Do you feel as deserving as the next person?
- Do you feel entitled to a good sex life?
- Do you think of yourself as a winner, rather than a loser?
- Do you describe yourself in glowing terms?
- Do you speak up for yourself?
- Are you proud of your successes?
- Do you surround yourself with upbeat friends who think highly of you?
- Do you think you have something to offer people?
- Do you have a thick skin and don't crumble if someone criticizes you?

SCORING:

For every yes answer, give yourself one point:

IF YOU SAID YES TO 0–4, you may be lacking in self-esteem and it's important to look at where you said no and work on your weak points. It can be affecting your sex life negatively.

IF YOU SAID YES TO 5–8, you have areas of strength and you may be on the right track, but you need to do some work. You have strong areas that are a great starting point to build on.

IF YOU SAID YES TO 9–12, you are in good shape. You still may want to take a look at the areas in which you are not feeling as confident, but you have pretty good self-esteem.

If you scored on the lower end, it's not hopeless. Building self-esteem isn't easy, and certainly doesn't come naturally. We are our worst critics, and need to learn how to become our own biggest fans. Check out these rules of thumb that sexually satisfied women follow to boost their morale, feel good about themselves, and let go of their insecurities.

Take risks in your everyday life.

What to do: Make choices without checking with a friend, partner, or spouse. It can be something simple, like calling a woman you meet at a dinner party and asking her to meet you for lunch. Or it can be something more complex, like changing jobs. People with low self-esteem are afraid to make a decision on their own. But if you take a chance and succeed, it's a guaranteed confidence-booster. The worst that can happen is that you fail, but you can't get anywhere if you don't try.

Confront your weaknesses head on.

What to do: Make a list of all the things you don't like about yourself. Don't hold back. The purpose isn't to make you feel bad; rather, it's to give you a sense of reality. For instance, if you write "I am a bad mother," are you really? You may work full-time, but your children are doing well, you spend time with your kids whenever you are home, you make sure they are well taken care of, arrange their child care and social activities—are you sure you're a bad mother? If you have low self-esteem and guilt on top of it, your life in general is going to suffer. So isolate what's causing you to feel poorly about yourself and address each issue one at a time.

Accept who you are.

What to do: Acknowledge your feelings, emotions, wants, and needs. Accept your limitations and what you can't change. Everyone has strengths and weaknesses, it's normal. Maybe you prefer to socialize with one good friend at a time instead of a large crowd. Some people are more comfortable in smaller groups. That's not necessarily a bad thing.

Perhaps you aren't a great athlete or musician. So what if you can't run a marathon or become a concert pianist? Neither can millions of others.

Get to the root of the problem.

What to do: Be it poor self-esteem, body image, or lack of self-worth, try to think about where these feelings may be coming from. Did you feel neglected growing up? Did your parents divorce when you were young? Did your siblings outshine you? Were your parents often critical of you? Were you a poor student no matter how hard you tried? Maybe even confronting your mother and father will help. Perhaps a close friend can help you get a grip on your past. If you have deep issues, talk to a therapist.

Think positively.

What to do: Thinking positively will help you *be* positive. Make a list of your attributes and what you like about yourself. Celebrate what you've done well. Take time to pat yourself on the back. Nothing is meaningless. Write down what you like about your body. This will take the focus off the negative. Laure Redmond, author of *Feel Good Naked*, suggests writing yourself a love letter once a month as a confidence booster. She says it will gradually, and hopefully permanently, shift your focus from self-criticism to love and acceptance.

Be assertive.

What to do: Once you have accepted and/or forgiven yourself and those who have damaged your self-esteem, move on. Venture out on challenges you have been putting off for fear of failure. Start that new business you have been dreaming about, call that old boyfriend you have been hankering to contact, go back to school and take those classes you need to further your education, take that vacation you have been yearning to go on, or invite that new neighbor over for tea.

Surround yourself with positive people.

What to do: Cultivate relationships with those who make you feel good about yourself. Avoid people who are judgmental and critical. Stay away from pessimists.

Keep in mind there are no simple solutions to building self-esteem; a therapist may be necessary to help you work toward self-acceptance. A therapist will point out where you are being too hard on yourself, give you a sense of reality, and help you get rid of any negative voices that may be speaking inside your head.

> **Women with a positive body image were more sexually satisfied and placed more importance on sexual satisfaction.**

FEELING GOOD NAKED

Are you obsessed with your body's shape? Do you think you are too fat, too tall, or too short? Do you fret about the size of your breasts? Are you uncomfortable with your nose, eyes, or facial features? Do you fear your stomach and thighs are too flabby? Are you preoccupied with the "perfect body" portrayed on television, in advertising, and in films? If so, you are among the bevy of women who struggle with their body image.

But take heed: Believing your body is never good enough can only hurt you, including in the bedroom. Dissatisfaction with your physical appearance can affect how you relate to your partner. And a negative body image can interfere with sexual pleasure. If you are hung up on your cellulite, it's hard to relax enough to sexually respond. It's tough to feel completely comfortable making love when you have a distorted body image. If you are busy hiding under the covers, you are not likely to try a sexual position that leaves your belly and thighs in full view. *The Journal of Sex Research* reported that approximately one-third of female college students were self-conscious about their body image during physical intimacy with a heterosexual partner.

Unfortunately, many women have unrealistic expectations about what they should look like. They have a distorted view of their own figure as well as the so-called ideal body shape. But they may be just the right size according to medical guidelines for height and weight. Laure Redmond points out in her book *Feel Good Naked* that Marilyn Monroe was actually a size fourteen.

Unrealistic expectations taken to the extreme can result in a condition called body dysmorphic disorder, which is a preoccupation with an imagined or minor physical defect. People who have this disorder see themselves as ugly, grotesque, or misshapen. This can lead to eating disorders and can have sexual and social ramifications because they see themselves as so profoundly flawed that they won't let anyone near them. It can ruin people's lives. They see themselves as different from everyone else, although they very rarely look abnormal.

Negative feelings about your body can have various causes, including:

Parental influence. While you were growing up, your parents didn't give positive feedback about your body and/or placed a huge emphasis on physical appearance. That can only lead to trouble, since so few of us can live up to those expectations.

Parents' obsession with weight. Your parents were constantly dieting and watching their weight, placing a large importance on being thin.

Childhood experiences. You heard derogatory comments growing up. Studies have shown that good-looking children tend to develop more self-confidence and have higher self-esteem than those perceived as less attractive. Making remarks like "My, she's a chubby one, isn't she?" or telling a young girl she is "interesting looking" or "you look just like your father" can prove harmful to her sense of feminine beauty.

Emotional, physical, or sexual abuse. Unwanted or inappropriate sexual attention can be associated with feeling bad and unworthy. Sexual abuse survivors can feel alienated from their bodies, deeming their bodies dirty, because that is the source of their pain and anxiety.

Peer rejection. Being ostracized as a child by your peers, or taunted for being too tall, overweight, wearing glasses, or having a big nose, can lead to adult consequences.

Social demand for the perfect body. You want to look like TV and film stars but don't. The media bombards us with messages that say a thin body is enviable. For women who feel they don't measure up, this can lead to eating disorders, such as anorexia and bulimia. In their book *Taking Charge of My Mind and Body*, Gladys Folkers and Jeanne Engelmann point out that many girls believe that living up to society's ideal of beauty is necessary to succeed, be popular, have friends, and attract boys.

Messages from lovers. Your partner makes unflattering remarks about your appearance. A lover can damage your body image with just one comment. We are extremely vulnerable when it comes to the impressions our lovers have of our bodies. Whether it's mentioning you need to lose or gain weight, exercise more, etcetera, it can shake confidence. Also, during an argument, criticism about your body is hard to forget.

We found that sexually satisfied women feel desirable naked no matter what they look like, and don't allow physical flaws to get in the way of passionate lovemaking. But don't despair; there are ways to improve your body image. Remember, the aim isn't to pose for *Playboy*, it's to change your self-perception and like the reflection that you see in the mirror. Here are some strategies for learning to love your body. Soon you'll be stripping down to the skin with all the lights on.

Mirror, Mirror on the Wall

You need to learn to love the image in the mirror—even with the bumps, pimples, dimples. Concentrate on your fabulous attributes. We all have some part of our body that makes us cringe. But think about the good parts. Maybe your hips are wide but your stomach is flat. Maybe your nose is large but you have a beautiful complexion. While we can all make the most with what we have, there are certain aspects of our bodies, no matter how much we diet or exercise, that we won't be able to alter. Heredity plays a big role in our body's shape and we can't change that. Michele Weiner Davis, in her book *The Sex-Starved Marriage*, says to focus on your good qualities and find ways to flaunt them.

Hello! Wake-Up Call!

Don't try to meet unrealistic body ideals the media portrays. It's not possible. According to the National Women's Health Resource Center, fashion models weigh 23 percent less than the average female. And don't obsess about your weight. Throw out the scale if you have to. No one should weigh themselves more than once a week. The scale is about numbers and has little to do with how you look.

You Can't Stop the Clock
So Stop Trying

Wrinkles are a natural part of life, but don't be afraid to take advantage of modern cosmetic medicine. As we get older, signs of aging surface. Some women are content living with the natural aging process and others are not. This varies greatly among sexually satisfied women. Making changes is all about personal choice. There is nothing shameful about wanting to enhance your youthful appearance, and there is nothing shameful about getting old gracefully. But if you are considering botox, collagen, or any form of plastic surgery, you need to question your motives. Are you doing it for yourself or for your partner? Are you hoping that changing your body will change your relationship? Are you looking for a quick fix to some other problem in your life? Before going under the knife you need to question your motives.

Berman Footnote

Although a positive body image is unequivocally essential for emotional and sexual well-being, you can't bury your head in the sand. If you just had a baby and you can't shed those extra pounds, or your baby is now twenty-five years old but each year the pounds just kept creeping up on you, you may be heavier than you want. If so, your sex life can suffer. It's not uncommon to pull back from intimate encounters if you are feeling fat and unattractive. It's also a fallacy to believe your partner will desire you unconditionally, and that the physical attraction should run so deep it doesn't matter if you gain forty or fifty pounds. That very well may be the case, and it's okay to expect your partner to love you no matter what, but it's unrealistic to assume he (or she) will be sexually attracted to you if your body has drastically changed. There are medical consequences from being overweight, too, as obesity leads to numerous health problems, including heart disease, diabetes, hypertension, and much more.

We all know that losing weight is not easy, and there are many reasons women have trouble shedding pounds, no matter how restricted their diet and how disciplined they are. As women age, their metabolism changes and staying thin is an uphill battle. Heredity plays a big part in your shape, too. You can't change your genes. Certainly not all women should strive for a slender body, as many different kinds of body types are sensual. If your partner knows you are invested in your appearance, it should make a difference in how he perceives you, regardless of what you weigh.

EVERY ROSE HAS ITS THORN: GENITAL SELF-ESTEEM

Women need to feel good about their genitals. Yes, every now and then a yeast infection will crop up, or a discharge or something unpleasant. But overall, you need to accept the way your genitals look, smell, and feel. Be proud of the female body's reproductive system and the ability to bear a child. Genital image is an important component of female sexuality.

Just as women have a hard time trying to live up to the perfect body image portrayed on TV, they have a hard time living up to the perfect genital image shown in magazines like *Playboy*. Most women aren't a size two with a flawless shape, and most women don't have perfectly shaped genitals. Your sexual anatomy may not be the shape or size you perceive as normal, but it doesn't mean there is anything wrong with you. In our experience, we have found a correlation between low genital self-image and low desire.

Pick up any number of popular magazines and you are bound to find articles on body image, but what about genital image? It's been underrepresented in the literature, but it shouldn't be. A woman's sex life can suffer if she feels negatively about her sexual organs.

Not too long ago we conducted a study looking at thirty-one patients with sexual dysfunction to determine if there is a relationship between genital image and sexual function complaints. We found that positive genital image was associated with higher sexual desire, although not with arousal, lubrication, orgasm, or satisfaction. A woman who feels confident about her genitals and is not ashamed of them is more likely to be sexually active.

The Fountain of Youth:
Eve's Story

By the time Eve was forty-five years old, she had almost every plastic surgery procedure imaginable. When she went to her high school reunion, even her closest friends from childhood hardly recognized her. "It's almost as if she is addicted to getting cosmetic work done," says Rosalie, a former classmate. "If she hadn't come up to me, I would have never known it was she." People who knew Eve well said she hated getting older, was unhappy with the way she looked, and felt she wasn't sexy enough for her husband.

Like Eve, there are people who visit the dermatologist or plastic surgeon as often as some of us visit the hairdresser. But while this is not the norm, and it's possible to overdo it, it's no longer unusual to improve your looks with the help of a medical specialist. A couple of decades ago it was mostly film and television celebrities who underwent nips and tucks. Now plastic surgery has gone mainstream, and working women and stay-at-home moms are going under the knife or needle. In fact, nowadays most of us know someone who has undergone some sort of cosmetic alteration. Whether it's a face-lift, botox, liposuction, or dental veneers, getting work done on your face or body has become much more common.

It's easy to get caught up in the hype. Consider the ABC-TV show *Extreme Makeover*. Women with facial or bodily defects, crooked teeth, who show signs of aging or who have unattractive features, are becoming Cinderellas on the air. After undergoing various procedures they are transformed into ravishing beauties. This feeds into many women's fantasies (and men's, too) of looking younger, prettier, and sexier.

For a long time women have struggled with obtaining an unrealistic ideal of what we see in the airbrushed pictures on the covers of magazines. But now there are more mechanisms than ever to achieve that.

As women age, they become preoccupied with having a youthful, sensual appearance. The numbers tell the story. According to the American Society of Plastic Surgeons, in 2003 more than 8.7 million cosmetic plastic surgery procedures were performed by ASPS members. This is up 32 percent from 2002, and includes face-lifts (lifting sagging facial skin and jowls), tummy tucks (removing excess fat from the abdomen), liposuction (removing fat deposits), eyelid surgery (fixing drooping eyelids), and breast lifts (reshaping and raising sagging breasts). Minimally invasive procedures are up 43 percent from 2002, and they include injections of botox, which is a botulism toxin (eliminating facial lines or wrinkles), chemical peels (restoring blemished and wrinkled skin with a chemical solution), dermabrasion (scraping the top layers of skin), laser hair removal, and collagen injections (adding fullness to the lips).

Unfortunately, in our society, the more youthful a woman looks, the more attractive she is considered. Throughout evolution, bright eyes, smooth skin, a clear complexion, and a symmetrical face were all signs of a woman's fertility and health. These are still signs of beauty today.

Anthropologist Helen Fisher, author of *The First Sex*, says in many cultures women become more powerful after menopause. "They don't have to keep trying to look like they are twenty-one in order to sustain the sexual power of a young girl," she says. In our country, women often lose power as they age and are considered less attractive, therefore we go to great lengths to alter our appearance.

There are different schools of thought related to cosmetic surgery, and we believe there is no clear right or wrong. Some mental health experts argue that propagating false expectations about the outcome of plastic surgery can lead women to fall prey to unrealistic ideals. It gives the message that unless we are complete perfection we are not good or sensual enough. Rather than seeing ourselves as getting more wrinkles, we should see ourselves as getting wiser. We should not allow ourselves to be manipulated into believing cosmetic surgery is the only way to get ahead. If a woman chooses to have work done in order to feel more sexual, she may be disappointed with the effect.

We see women every day in our practices who are not happy with their bodies. They are embarrassed and complain about being fat, are uptight having sex or letting their partners see them naked. Some undergo plastic surgery and some don't. We support whatever decision they make. If a woman doesn't feel good about a part of her body or face to the point that it affects her self-esteem, then it may be perfectly reasonable to do something about it.

But beauty is only skin deep. It must be recognized that making yourself more beautiful on the outside won't automatically change the way you feel about yourself on the inside. If a woman suffers from self-esteem issues, altering her face won't change the way she feels about herself. Surgical alterations are not going to solve problems, and looking stunning doesn't automatically guarantee a better sex life. Cosmetic surgery isn't likely to rid a woman of her sexual inhibitions, especially if they are deeply rooted. A physical makeover won't necessarily act as an emotional or psychological makeover.

Women who undergo cosmetic alterations and women who are comfortable with the natural aging process can all have a satisfying sex life. Whether a woman celebrates her body on her own, through therapy, or as a result of plastic surgery, it doesn't make a difference. Feeling good about your body no matter how you got there translates into having a better sex life.

SOCCER FIELD OR WALL STREET?

How does working or staying at home play a role in a woman's sexual satisfaction? When a woman spreads herself too thin it leaves little time or energy for a fulfilling sex life. The hardest of all is balancing a full-time job with full responsibility for the kids. Women who try to do both pay a hefty price. They are exhausted, overwrought, too tired for sex, and yes, let's not forget the guilt. They are harder on themselves when it comes to mothering and they feel guilty about not doing so-called maternal tasks. They are ashamed to bring store-bought cookies to the class potluck supper instead of baking. They feel at fault if they can't be the parental chaperone on the class trip. But women who are most successful in balancing both understand that sometimes you have to cut corners; you may have to be late for work or to the school play, but it is the only way to survive the emotional stress.

There is a misconception that women who stay home don't have any stress. The fact is, they do. They can feel wrong about staying home, and are often looked down upon by their working peers. They are surrounded by kids all day and lacking in adult conversation. Since there are no clear-cut hours or a set lunch break, they are unable to carve out time for themselves. A working woman may be too exhausted to have sex, but the stay-at-home mom is just as drained.

The good news is many mothers' expectations are changing. A decade earlier women thought they could, and should, do it all—work, take care of the kids, and have an active social life. But being on the fast track at work can take away from quantity and quality time with the kids, let alone with your husband or partner or even yourself. Therefore, many mothers who are financially secure and don't need the dual family income have chosen to rear their children full-time, putting their careers temporarily aside. According to the Census Bureau in 2002, of the 41.8 million kids under fifteen who lived with two parents, more than 25 percent had mothers who stayed home. That was up from 1994.

Of course, staying at home is not an option for many moms, either because they are single or because the family requires a second income to cover the cost of education, the mortgage, and living expenses. Middle-class expenses are not what they used to be—private schools, sporting equipment, dental braces, summer camps, and music lessons are all commonplace for many American families. Colleges and universities can run $100,000 and upward for a four-year degree.

The key for both working mothers and stay-at-home moms, whether they spend their days at the office or at home by choice or necessity, is having some "me" time. We may feel depressed, stressed, tired, sick, but we ignore our ailments and woes to take care of our families. We have a reservoir of energy in our bodies, but if we don't keep that reservoir full or replenished, we slowly go to empty, which leaves no sexual energy. In order to be more inspired sexually, it's important to spend more time by and for yourself.

ANXIETY AND DEPRESSION: WALKING ON THE EDGE

Depression affects all areas of a person's life and is as real an illness as cancer or heart disease. People who are depressed usually describe a feeling of hopelessness, worthlessness, and inadequacy. When a person is depressed, sex is one of the last things on his or her mind. Depending on the degree of depression, whether it's mild or severe, sufferers can find it hard to get out of bed in the morning, let alone become sexually intimate. Chronic depression can cause low energy, decreased libido, and a loss of interest in doing anything pleasurable.

> Our survey results indicated that women with mental health problems were less sexually satisfied.

Women are at a greater risk for depression than men. It may have to do with the additional stresses that they are up against at work and at home. Many women have full-time jobs and the sole responsibility for their children. But whatever the cause, depressive episodes over a long period of time can affect hormone levels in the body that ultimately lead to depression.

How do you know if you are depressed? Everyone has days when they feel blah. But depression isn't just being a little blue or sad. It's an unrelenting feeling of hopelessness. Symptoms of clinical depression include:

- **Change in sleep patterns, either sleeping too much or suffering from insomnia**
- **Change in eating habits, either overeating or experiencing diminished appetite**
- **Change in the joy of life, not feeling motivated to have fun**
- **Having trouble concentrating**
- **Feeling sad, worthless, isolated**
- **Feeling hopeless about the future**
- **Suicidal thoughts**

It's not always clear at what point you should seek medical attention. But if you are having trouble functioning or don't have the energy or the desire to take part in activities you once liked, it's time to talk to your doctor. It is also possible that these symptoms mean something is physically wrong.

The good news is that depression is highly treatable with either talk therapy or antidepressants, or a combination of the two. Antidepressants usually take about four to six weeks to take effect and help patients get back to living their lives. They work by regulating chemicals in the brain called neurotransmitters. Researchers believe that depressed people have an imbalance of certain neurotransmitters in the brain, in particular serotonin and norepinephrine. The most common antidepressants act by increasing the level of these neurotransmitters.

Fortunately, there are more than a dozen prescription antidepressant medications on the market that do this. The bad news, however, is that while side effects are few, the most common potential side effects are lack of libido and lowered sexual sensation. In fact, the most commonly prescribed medications for depression—called SSRIs (selective serotonin reuptake inhibitors)—such as Prozac, Zoloft, and Paxil can cause a decline in sexual functioning. When this happens, sexual desire may diminish, genital sensation is lowered, and it's harder to reach orgasm. So, unfortunately, some women successfully alleviate their symptoms of depression only to find they have no libido.

> Antidepressant use is related to less sexual satisfaction.

This is not an easy dilemma to solve. Doesn't seem just, does it? But treatment shouldn't be compromised when it interferes with sexual functioning; instead, solutions need to be explored. Patients can talk to their prescribing physician about experimenting with lower doses, or perhaps trying another medication with hopes of lowering the sexual side effects. Some women have had success switching to Wellbutrin or combining it with other antidepressants. A woman may ultimately need to incorporate vibrators or more foreplay into her sex life if there is a response problem. There is also evidence that a low-dose testosterone cream can improve mood and libido.

Some studies have found that Viagra helps to counteract negative sexual side effects in women who are taking SSRIs. We participated in a twelve-week study looking at the effectiveness of sildenafil (Viagra) in 202 postmenopausal or posthysterectomized women with female sexual arousal disorder. The women who took Viagra reported better overall sexual satisfaction as opposed to the women who took the placebo. It seems that Viagra was well tolerated and increased the blood flow to the genitalia.

As mentioned above, medication plays a large role in treating depression, and is often used in conjunction with psychotherapy to help understand the root of the problem and to change the negative thought process. Medication can relieve the depression but not the issues causing it in the first place. Once the medication has been stopped, the depression may return if the issues causing the depression haven't improved. Of course, when the depression is caused by a chemical imbalance, talk therapy doesn't help.

The hope is that eventually the medication will be able to be discontinued. But for women who can't tolerate stopping, there are ways around the sexual side effects if you're willing to experiment and find what works for you.

Anxiety

Feeling anxious isn't unusual. We all have worries that make us feel on edge. But when our anxiety lingers and interferes with our daily functioning, it's time to seek professional help. There are different kinds of anxieties:

> **PANIC ATTACKS.** Sudden feeling of terror accompanied by trembling, racing heart, sweatiness, and even nausea and dizziness.

> **PHOBIAS.** Irrational fears and intense panic that can cause heart palpitations and light-headedness when faced with heights, animals, closed spaces, open spaces, leaving the house, speaking in public, and more. It can become very limiting and isolating, making it difficult to interact with others.

> **GENERALIZED ANXIETY DISORDER.** Nonstop free-floating worries about health, children, spouse, parents, work, or money. Dwelling on the worst-case scenario and possible catastrophes.

If you are struggling with anxiety, sex is probably not the first thing on your mind. When someone is anxious, even if they are having sex, they may have a hard time focusing. For some, sex itself is a trigger for anxiety. They are self-conscious about their bodies and want to run and hide when their partners see them without their clothes on. Or they have performance anxiety, afraid they won't be able to sexually satisfy or be satisfied. Some women become distressed when they start to sexually respond because, when they are stimulated, they feel they are losing control and that scares them.

If anxiety is getting the best of you, taking over your life, if you can't engage in the activities you once did and are having trouble sleeping, eating, and enjoying a full sex life, talk to your doctor.

A FRIEND IN NEED IS A FRIEND INDEED: IMPORTANCE OF SOCIAL SUPPORT

Believe it or not, having a network of friends can improve your sex life. We found that sexually satisfied women have a network of companions other than, and along with, their mate, which in turn helps their sex life for the following reasons:

- When they spend time with their female friends it makes them feel more feminine and helps them reconnect as a woman.
- The woman-to-woman time can foster independence, relaxation, and just plain fun.
- Sharing information about their sexual problems, trouble-shooting, and offering tips can be therapeutic. It lets them know they are not alone, that others have the same sexual problems.

Socializing with Your Mate Can Also Be Just What the Doctor Ordered

- Going out with couples deflects some of the pressure of always trying to make conversation. It's also a way to avoid personal conflict. Therefore, if you are experiencing marital strife and need a breather in order to calm down and get your sex life back on track, being out with friends can be a welcome break. Laughing and having a great night out with other couples can spill over to enjoyment in the bedroom.

- Having a time-out with friends is a bonding experience that can inspire a sexual energy. Seeing a steamy, romantic movie with a group of friends and talking about it over dinner can be an inspiration for later in the evening.

Social support is a key element in gaining emotional health as well. Having solid friendships, someone with whom you can discuss your problems, can help guard against stress and anxiety. If a woman is isolated and doesn't have anyone to talk to, or to help her with everyday demands, it takes an emotional toll.

If you feel the need to increase your social ties, consider initiating a relationship with your neighbor, or mothers at your child's school, or expanding your social network by joining a group or volunteering in the community.

BOTTOM LINE

Our survey showed that women who enjoy life are the ones who are most content with their sex lives. Emotional well-being and sexual satisfaction go hand in hand, so use the tips you learned in this chapter to put the lust back into your life and to feel better overall. It will pay off and you deserve it. The happier you are with yourself, the happier you'll be in bed.

Relationship
Health

The Emotional
Connection

I n this chapter we focus on the fundamentals of a sexual relationship: meeting a mate, falling in love, the initial infatuation, and formation of a long-term commitment and bond. Sexually satisfied women report that they cherish the intimacy and emotional connection in their relationship. For women, the more attentive and invested the partner

---

FINDINGS FROM THE WOMEN'S
SEXUAL SATISFACTION SURVEY

Sexually satisfied women say:

- There is a strong relationship between intimacy, communication, and sexual satisfaction.
- Size matters: Sexually satisfied women are more likely to be satisfied if their partner has a large penis.

---

is in the relationship, the more secure she feels, and ultimately the more responsive she will be sexually.

THAT AGE-OLD QUESTION

Okay, before we talk about intimacy, sex appeal, and all the components that go along with a healthy relationship, we thought we would cut right to the chase: Does size matter? It's what everyone wants to know! In our study, women who described their partners as having a larger penis were more likely to be satisfied. In terms of how the guys measured up: 3 percent of women described their partner's penis as small or very small, 64 percent said average, and 39 percent said large to very large.

So, does size matter? The answer is yes. Our findings show sexually satisfied women say it makes a difference. But even if your partner has a small-sized penis, you can have as much fun in bed and be as connected and intimate as you would with a man with a larger penis. It's true that a larger penis can lead to enhanced "sensations" of pleasure, but it is not required.

It's a myth that a bigger penis makes a man more masculine. What makes a man more masculine is his ability to be emotionally supportive and having a strong character and strong values. And the ability to biologically father a child has little to do with penis size.

What do you do if you feel your partner's penis is too small or too large? Following are some tips.

If the penis is on the smaller size, consider these tips:

The pregame show.
What to do: Focus more on foreplay as the source of your sexual release than on actual intercourse. Not that you can't have intercourse, just make sure you get the stimulation you need in other ways.

Trial run.
What to do: Experiment with different positions. For some women there are limitations if a man has a shorter penis. You may not be able to do it from behind, or in different positions that require more length. You may have to vary the kind of positions that you engage in.

Changing gears.
What to do: Focus on the fact that clitoral stimulation is the primary way that most women reach orgasm. Concentrate on positions that optimize clitoral stimulation.

Look beyond.
What to do: Strengthen other aspects of the sexual encounter. Many men who have gone through life with a smaller penis have learned to compensate and will have gained skills in oral sex and manual stimulation. Enjoy those skills and enjoy the part of the sexual relationship that works well.

The big squeeze.

What to do: Optimize your use of the pelvic-floor muscles during intercourse. The vagina is a potential space, so it can squeeze around a tampon or loosen up enough for a baby to pass through. We have the capacity to change the size of our vagina during a sexual encounter by using the pelvic muscles. Doing Kegel exercises will help strengthen your pelvic-floor muscles, which play a vital role in arousal and climax (as well as controlling urinary continence). The more toned your pelvic muscles are, the more sexual satisfaction you can achieve.

What to do if the penis is too large:

Look beyond.

What to do: If it's too large to feel enjoyable, you may need to use other kinds of sexual stimulation for your sexual pleasure and release.

Loosen up.

What to do: Sometimes, when you relax the pelvic-floor muscles, you can hold the larger penis.

Get wet.

What to do: Use lubricants.

Fall short.

What to do: Don't insert the penis all the way.

Keep it simple.

What to do: Avoid any complicated positions that are painful or require deep thrusting.

Berman Footnote

If your partner's penis is indeed too small, chances are he has faced stumbling blocks or has dealt with locker-room ridicule. Whatever the penis size may be, always focus on the positive and concentrate on what works best. For example, if it's not working in a certain position you will want to avoid highlighting his insufficiencies. For example, instead of saying "Your penis is too small to do it in that position," you might say "It feels really good when we do it in this position and I really love it, can we do more of that?" Your partner may be aware of your motives, but he will appreciate your consideration and candor. What really matters in the end is that you love him and are attracted to him.

SEX APPEAL: WHAT DRAWS US TO THE OPPOSITE SEX?

All right, now that we have that burning question about penis size out of the way, we can get on with the nitty-gritty of a relationship.

Ever meet someone for the first time and think they aren't very good-looking, but when you get to know them, the appeal starts to grow? While physical attraction is extremely important in a relationship, it may not happen immediately. With women in particular, attraction to a partner is not all about physical appearance. If a partner has a sense of humor, is dependable, trustworthy, interesting, and successful, it's often okay if he or she doesn't meet the classic standards of beauty. There needs to be more than just physical chemistry to keep the sparks flying. Looks typically fade over time, and if there is no intimacy and trust, the relationship will start to suffer.

What attracts one person to another is in part related to our evolutionary history. Males are evolutionarily programmed to look for signs of fertility in potential mates in order to ensure their ability to pass on their genes. For example, big breasts and hips are important attraction cues for some men, as they are signs of fertility. Men want someone younger in her reproductive years, with a robust body, complete with "child-bearing hips," indicating an ability to bear children. Women in ancient times were considered more attractive if their eyes were bright and their skin was clear, as they were signs of good health. If the face and features were symmetrical, it was a sign of a good gene pool.

Women, on the other hand, looked not only for reproductive viability and good health, but also for someone strong and with social status. They wanted a mate who could survive and provide important resources, a man with strength and the power to protect who was also a good hunter and could supply food. In Helen Fisher's *Why We Love: The Nature and Chemistry of Romantic Love*, she proposes that monogamy is a contract between men and women. A woman committed her social and marital life to one male partner so that he would assume the children he was supporting were his. In return he made a commitment of monogamy to her from the standpoint of supporting her, bringing her meat and resources.

We see similarities today—young, attractive, reproductively viable women on the arms of older wealthy men. The men may not be particularly handsome, but they have power and status and therefore are attractive as partners.

We see older men who leave their wives for younger, sometimes more alluring women. According to Dr. Ellen Haimoff, New York City eating disorders specialist, bulimia and anorexia are on the rise in middle-aged women. These women feel if they are not thin enough or desirable enough, their partners will abandon them. Dr. Haimoff, who says that about 30 percent of her practice consists of women over age thirty-five, finds that the baby boomers want to look young, thin, and beautiful, and this can exert a tremendous pressure to maintain the look of a reproductively viable thirty-year-old. They are suddenly dealing with hormonal issues, marital strife, empty nest syndrome, the death of a parent, and fear of divorce. They worry their husbands or partners might leave them for more youthful versions of themselves, a worry that is either imagined or real. Many become exercise addicts, consumed with going to the gym.

But keep in mind and take to heart that if your relationship is healthy and both partners are satisfied, it is unlikely that he'll stray. This is not to say that making him happy should become a full-time job, but relationships do require work, and it's important not to become complacent or passive in the relationship.

While it was once rare to see older women on the arms of attractive younger men, we are seeing more of it, especially with the baby boomer women. It's not quite as shocking as it once was. Take high-profile couples like Demi Moore and Ashton Kutcher—people are saying good for her, as well as good for him. And it's not just Hollywood actresses linked to twenty-something hunks; lots of forty-something women are making a love connection with twenty- or thirty-something men.

But assuming you have been in a stable, passionate relationship, what happens if all of a sudden you realize you are no longer physically attracted to your partner? What can you do if the spark has gone out?

Get real. Before you end a perfectly good relationship and ditch someone you were physically attracted to at some point in time, make sure your expectations are realistic. Does this person look good for his or her age? Is he or she relatively fit? Or has he or she lost interest in their appearance? Ask yourself if this is more about you or the other person.

Look within. Is this about your self-esteem, in that you need a man or woman to look a certain way in order to feel good about yourself? If so, perhaps you should reevaluate your priorities.

Once you have ruled out any personal self-esteem issues and determined it's more about your partner than you, think about what you can do to regain that attraction. Consider these possibilities:

Think physical health. If it has to do with weight gain, explain you are concerned about his or her health and want to help. Offer to join in the effort to shed pounds. Suggest joining a health club or taking walks together.

Think mental health. If he or she seems depressed, is under undue stress, or is unhappy with life in general, it could affect any motivation to look good. Help him or her become aware of the symptoms in order to recognize there's a problem and get the therapeutic help needed. You can offer to find a good therapist and make the appointment, even go along. If there is any resistance, offer to make it a joint session. Sometimes your partner needs someone to help take the initiative. It's crucial for anyone who is depressed to get help because symptoms rarely improve on their own, and there is much more at risk than a little weight gain. Depression can lead to destructive behavior and even suicide.

Think floundering sex life. Maybe your partner's lack of motivation to take care of himself or herself is because things have started to fall apart for you both emotionally and sexually. Perhaps your partner is acting out because he or she is angry at you for not being interested in sex. Or maybe he or she isn't feeling romantic anymore because sex isn't happening.

Be blunt. Sometimes it gets to a point where you get turned off. Therefore say: "I love you, I care about you, I want you, and have always been attracted to you. But since you are not invested in your appearance, it's affecting how I feel about you sexually, and I don't want that to happen."

> **Women who had more intimacy with their partners were more sexually satisfied and placed more importance on sexual satisfaction.**

THE SEXUAL BOND

For sexually satisfied women, intimacy and closeness are the foundation for sexual satisfaction and sexual feelings. It's the commitment, security, affection, and caring that arouse women most.

Quality time, communication, feeling you are special, and believing your partner cares what you think and offers unconditional support go hand in hand with commitment. When there is doubt, sex can suffer.

The sexual bond for women usually begins outside of the bedroom. It's only when a solid comfort level, familiarity, and warmth have been established that a healthy relationship can develop.

MR. OR MRS. RIGHT

We all know that meeting a mate isn't always easy. In fact, with the demands we all face in everyday life, finding romance can be downright difficult. We are spending more hours at work, have less leisure time, and are getting married later. So where can a woman go to find a partner? It's not like the turn of the last century, when families relied on matchmakers to find spouses for their daughters, or the 1950s, when women met a partner in high school or college and had to get married in order to have sex. Today's matchmakers take the form of friends, organized trips for singles, wine tasting and cooking classes, health clubs, church or synagogue functions for singles, cafés, and, of course, the Internet.

In looking for a partner it's also very important for women to know what their priorities are in life as well as in their mate. What are the qualities and characteristics you want in a long-term partner? What do you value most? What areas are you willing or not willing to compromise on? It is helpful to write these things down on paper, and use them from time to time as a reference and reminder about what is important to you. It will help keep you on track in the difficult and cumbersome journey of finding a mate.

ONLINE DATING

Online dating is fast becoming one of the most popular ways to meet someone. According to the market research firm comScore Media Metrix, approximately forty million Americans a month visit the more than sixty websites that have some kind of dating personals. When twenty-nine-year-old Lauren broke up with her boyfriend of three years, she was out of circulation and hard pressed for where to find dates. Tired of the bar scene, she thought she'd try the Internet. "So many people are doing it, there is no stigma, and I thought I'd have nothing to lose," she says. "I was right—some of the guys were cute and smart. I've had many dates already, and wound up dating a couple of them for a while."

Many sites accommodate all age groups. Upon signing and paying a monthly fee, you build a profile anonymously, keeping your identity private. You may or may not scan in your photo. Prospects e-mail you, and the rest is up to your discretion. You also have the option of surfing the site and e-mailing any promising suitors.

There are many advantages to online dating—for instance, being anonymous allows you to create a relationship through e-mail before meeting. This way you can screen numerous potential matches, and it's a respectable way to meet someone. Still, there are pitfalls. Some people misrepresent themselves, some may be married, and some may have questionable backgrounds. Another problem: You may be looking for a long-term relationship but not everyone is seeking a love connection. One thing to bear in mind when it comes to online dating is that you need to be patient. This will take time and you will probably have to screen through a lot of Mr. Wrongs, go on a lot of dates, and drink a lot of coffee before you find Mr. Right. Most important is to be honest about yourself and what you are looking for. This is the perfect opportunity to cut to the chase.

PUTTING YOURSELF OUT THERE

There is, however, a risk when you meet someone blindly, without any personal references, so be cautious. In *Wired Not Weird: A Woman's Guide to Dating Online,* authors Christy Clement and Kay McLean warn that not everyone online is looking for love—some are predators looking for sex. Unsuspecting women, naive, innocent, and vulnerable, can easily fall prey. Even savvy women can get duped or exercise bad judgment. More often than not, the men will be normal, law-abiding citizens. But you never know for sure.

Here are some rules of caution for online dating:

No vital stats. To avoid any misconceptions, when describing yourself, limit physical descriptions to the basics—height, weight, coloring, etcetera. Overzealous descriptions of physique and physical attributes are inappropriate and a red flag, so beware.

Less is more. Don't give out any identifying information, such as your last name, address, where you work, or any personal information until after you meet and only after you have a fairly good idea the person is trustworthy and that you're interested.

Be suspicious. Before you spend time alone, which should never happen at the first meeting, check out where he works and verify he's telling the truth. Find out where he's from, where he went to school, etcetera. See if you know anyone in common and check the facts.

Rules of engagement. You should correspond for several weeks and talk on the phone at least twice before you meet in person; a telephone conversation can reveal discrepancies. Avoid people who are evasive or who don't answer your questions. In fact, if you don't get your simple questions answered during the first few weeks, stop writing.

Thanks, but no thanks. Once you put your profile and/or picture on a website, you are likely to get dozens of responses. If you find that a particular person isn't for you, then politely say it's not going to work out.

Stay in public places. For safety, it's always advisable to meet in a public place, like a bar or restaurant. Meeting at a quiet deserted place can be dangerous. And never meet for the first time at his house or apartment—that's looking for trouble. Don't go out solo until you have met in a public place at least three or four times.

Be e-mail savvy. Make sure your e-mail address doesn't spell out your name, don't use your work e-mail, and know how to block e-mails and blind copy.

Get a wingman. Consider telling the waitperson you are on a blind date in case anything suspicious occurs. Get a friend to come to the bar or restaurant to sit nearby. If that can't happen, make sure someone knows where you will be. Share everything you know about him.

Triple protection. Avoid getting in a car with him—either drive yourself or take a cab. Keep your cell phone with you in case of an emergency. Don't leave with him and walk down a secluded street. It's a good idea to check in with either a friend or family member during the evening.

Go with your gut. Trust your intuition before making a second date. Your gut is always right.

SPEED DATING

Another hot trend in finding romance is speed dating. It was originally started by a rabbi who wanted to unite Jewish singles in the hopes they would marry within their faith. But it caught on nondenominationally across the country and beyond. Here is how it works: An equal number of men and women are paired off for eight minutes. A bell rings and they switch chairs and partners. Pens and paper are supplied for note taking, and each person is given a scorecard to circle either yes (if they would like to see that person again) or no (if they did not feel a connection). At the end of the evening each person turns in his or her scorecard and e-mail address. The next day a list of all the people you matched with is e-mailed to you. From then on, the ball is in your court.

These quick encounters, which pretty much rely on first impressions and gut reactions, give the chance to either connect or bail. The downside is possibly passing up someone great.

Of course, the old-fashioned blind date is always a good way to meet a mate. This way you have the advantage of a mutual party in common, which lessens the usual risks. Don't be shy or afraid to ask friends and colleagues if they know someone who may be suitable for you. A potential mate could be an acquaintance, friend, or relative of a coworker, schoolmate, or business associate. And when you do get "fixed up," give it a chance. First impressions aren't always accurate.

TAKING THE LEAD

All right, now that you have met an appealing prospect, can you be the initiator? The answer is yes. The rules of dating have changed since the sexual revolution. In the beginning women had to sit passively and wait for a man to call them. Now, as part of our overall empowerment and assertiveness, women can and should be more proactive. Making the first move or pursuing a date is much more acceptable today. Perhaps that potential love interest may need a little push to get to know you, see your attributes firsthand, and get to appreciate your personality. You can be the one to size up the situation. If you feel you have made a connection but he or she doesn't call back, it's okay to phone him or her. Still, there is something to be said about playing a little hard to get. Many men like to be the pursuers and get turned off by a woman who is too pushy, aggressive, or desperate.

Taking the Lead:
Emily's Story

Emily, a twenty-seven-year-old writer, met David while she was a freshman in college; they were close friends but never dated. Emily started to feel attracted to David in a different way within the last few years and wasn't sure how to proceed. She began by giving David signs that she was interested. She invited him for dinner, then asked him to spend the weekend with her at her family's summer cottage. Eventually she was forthright in telling him she wasn't satisfied with just being platonic. They began going on dates and before long a romance developed. Last year, after five years of dating, they married.

But not everybody's story has a happy ending. What if he or she doesn't respond? How do you handle rejection? First of all, rejection happens to everyone, and if you make the first move, you need to be prepared that you can be hurt. Men have taken the risk throughout history. Anytime you take a risk in life it makes you stronger, even if you get turned down. If you are consistently rejected, however, you may want to take a look at your style. There may be something else going on.

In dating, the key is feeling good about yourself and making it clear through your actions and demeanor that you are happy, confident, and independent. You don't want to look or sound like a poor soul. Being desperate or needy isn't exactly a crowd-pleaser.

Check out these tricks of the trade to exude an air of confidence:

Play the part.

What to do: If you don't feel self-confident, try acting as if you are. Practicing self-assurance is the first step toward feeling it. Most of us have seen the women who keep men wrapped around their fingers. Men will do anything they want. What these women have in common is an air of self-assurance and confidence. They simply respect themselves and assume others will, too.

Get a hobby.

What to do: Having your own special interests always helps. If you don't have any hobbies or pastimes, and have no outside interests, you are much more likely to feel and appear needy. Not to mention that you'll likely give the impression that the person you end up with will be your whole life. The more independent and self-sufficient you are, the better you will fare. And if you have a variety of interests, it will expand your social network, giving you more opportunities to meet potential mates. If you don't have a particular hobby, consider getting a pet. A dog, cat, bird, even tropical fish can be an outside interest.

GIVE LOVE A CHANCE

While having "chemistry" with a partner is an essential part of making a connection, it's not the only factor. If you meet someone you have a lot in common with, and there is a little attraction but not a tremendous amount, you may want to give the person a chance. Often when someone has an endearing personality, physical attraction grows. In sorting out the pros and cons of forging ahead in a relationship, follow these rules:

- Make a list of all the characteristics you seek in a lifetime mate. Putting them down on paper can help clarify what's important to you. Do you want someone witty, attractive, or athletic? What about ambitious, motivated, or wealthy? Or maybe very intelligent, highly educated, and cultured? Write your preferences down in order of importance. Does this person fit the bill?

- If he or she has glaring or disagreeable qualities that you can't tolerate, you have a choice to either accept the imperfections or walk away. However, do not be unrealistic in your expectations. Nobody is perfect, and if you are looking for Mr. or Ms. Perfection, you might well be disappointed.

- If those flaws are dangerous or serious ones, such as being violent or a substance abuser, you should not continue with the relationship. If there are things you don't like, beware; don't expect to change someone to a new, improved version once you've got your paws on him or her.

- Once you do start to build a relationship, it's okay to discuss your feelings, but don't begin pressuring the other person about getting serious prematurely. That can scare anyone away.

WAKE UP AND SMELL THE REALITY

If your relationship isn't progressing, or your partner seems to be backing off, or he is making excuses why you can't be together or why he can't call, open your eyes to what may really be going on: He may be losing interest. Or, like that famous line in *Sex and the City*: "He's just not that into you!"

Let's face it, when your relationship is blossoming, you know it. In the book *He's Just Not That Into You: The No-Excuses Truth to Understanding Guys*, authors Greg Behrendt and Liz Tuccillo, who both worked on *Sex and the City*, warn women not to rationalize away poor behavior, to recognize negative signs, and to know when the relationship is going sour.

How can you tell if he *is* into you? If he actually does what he says he is going to, writes Behrendt and Tuccillo. What are some signs he *isn't* into you?

- He doesn't call when he says he is going to.
- He refuses to make a commitment.
- He constantly lets you down.
- He doesn't make you feel good about yourself.
- He says he wants to date others.
- He is having sex with other women besides you.
- He is not willing to talk about the relationship.
- He says he is not anywhere near ready for marriage.

The bottom line: If you have given the relationship your all and he isn't responding, it's time to move on.

THE HONEYMOON STAGE AND AFTER

Let's say your relationship is going well, you think you have found your soul mate, and the feeling is mutual. Your emotions are running high. You have built a foundation for a potential lasting love. But a solid relationship passes through many stages, from infatuation to contentment and a more mature love. While the honeymoon doesn't last forever, the best is yet to come. Here is what you can expect:

Seeing Fireworks:
The Infatuation Stage

You have recently met and are filled with euphoria, intensity, and passion. You are blissfully happy, there is an element of mystery, you can't keep your hands off each other, lust is constant, and you have sex all the time. You are on a constant high. Unfortunately, you can't sustain yourself in the infatuation stage for very long because it's likely your obsession with one another would eventually interfere with everyday functioning. Nature works in a way that allows familiarity to build in a relationship and the infatuation stage eventually ends—for everyone.

But beware, however, of the noncommittal "infatuation junkie." This is someone who goes from relationship to relationship, and as soon as it turns into something deeper, he (or she) jumps ship. He becomes bored, or finds the increased intimacy too scary, or is afraid of opening his heart for fear of getting hurt. This may not even be conscious. The infatuation stage is safe, sexy, fun, and too early to worry or plan for the future.

How do you know if you or your partner is an infatuation junkie? These are the signs:

- **Every three to six months you are on to a new partner.**
- **You can't stand to be without a sexual partner.**
- **After a period of time boredom sets in.**
- **You are attracted to people who are unavailable or married.**

If this sounds familiar, take a second look. If you are dating someone like this, it's unlikely it will go much farther without some serious soul searching on his part. If it's you who have these characteristics, it's no wonder you haven't settled down yet. It's not that you can't find love that lasts, it's that you can't seem to move on from infatuation to attachment. Take a good look at what you are afraid of and give love a try . . . you may enjoy the quieter kind just as much. If it's just too scary or too uncomfortable, it might be time to seek professional help to get to the bottom of your fears and resolve them.

He's a Keeper:
The Attachment Phase

You have moved down to earth—your intensity has slowed down. But while that dreamy love may have waned, there is security, comfort, and contentment. It's a deeper kind of love, says Helen Fisher in her book *Anatomy of Love*, this sensation called attachment saturates the mind. Fisher describes this stage as the most elegant of human feelings.

What's Love Got to Do with It?

Love has become routine and you may even take your partner for granted at times. Familiarity sets in, and the novelty of being excited whenever you are together has worn off. But that's normal and it doesn't mean you have fallen out of love. So don't break it off or be discouraged. It doesn't mean that the relationship is stale, just different. It's okay if your heart no longer beats fast when he walks in the door. Just keep the passion going, foster the love, and enjoy the emotional closeness.

Resting on Your Laurels:
Contentment

Love is here to stay. Sparks might not be flying, but the passion is solid and strong. You are friends as well as lovers, you are secure and comfortable. You have a bond that is hard to break. Enjoy and cherish it. Sex doesn't have to be old hat—keep it exciting and don't stop trying new ways to make love.

TAKING THE STABLE RELATIONSHIP INTO THE BEDROOM

Indeed, there is a difference between what men and women want or need sexually. Men tend to be ready to move from foreplay to intercourse quicker; they also seem to want more direct genital stimulation sooner. What a lot of couples don't realize is they can meet each other's needs at the same time. During foreplay, the male partner can meet the woman's erotic needs by slowly kissing her neck, shoulders, and other erogenous zones prior to going directly to the genitals. While the man is stimulating her erogenous zones, she can be stimulating his genitals directly, and they both are having their sexual needs met.

Once the arousal occurs, they are often on a much more even plane. It's the same with different sexual positions. Your partner may like one position that you are just okay with, and he may feel the same about your favorite position. It works best to take turns. You don't have to be at the same pace in terms of your arousal process, nor at the same pace with your orgasm. Consider getting into your favorite position and focusing on your pleasure, so that he won't reach orgasm too soon. This allows you to have one, too.

When trying to get your sexual needs across, it's important to focus on the positive. Try "I" statements: "I would love it if we could . . ." "It feels great to me when we . . ." "I would love if we could do more . . ." Introduce it outside the bedroom first. For example, "Last night was really amazing, I enjoyed it so much I was thinking next time I want to try . . ." When you are in the midst of a sexual situation it can be a bit intimidating sometimes for the partner, so don't focus on the negative. If there is something that your partner is doing wrong, you don't want to say: "Don't do that, I don't like it." Instead, you want to say: "You know what I like even more than that . . ." and give them an alternative that you may enjoy.

SAYING NO TO SEX

No matter how explosive your sex life, what erotic games you play or fantasies you act out, there is bound to be a time when you or your partner will not be in the mood for sex. Perhaps you are sick, angry with your partner, or have something going on emotionally. Maybe there is a movie you want to see on TV, or you want to do the laundry. It could be that you are exhausted and want to get a good night's sleep. It's normal and a part of life. It's to be expected. You don't have to say yes to sex all the time.

On the other hand, you shouldn't say no too quickly or too frequently. You also need to be aware of what saying no does to your partner emotionally. Here are some rules about saying no to sex:

Be sensitive. Too many no's can make your partner feel abandoned, rejected, and unattractive. So if you want to hold back, it is important that you do it gently.

Don't place blame. Tell your partner it's not about him or her; it's about you. Explain that you are not feeling well, or discuss the reason why you are not in the mood. Make a date to have sex—and keep it.

Power struggle. It's never okay to say no if it's about manipulation and power. Withholding sex should not be used as punishment or a means of getting what you want.

Using Sex for Power:
Nancy's Story

Nancy, in her early thirties, decided to withhold her body as a way of getting back at her boyfriend, Jay. He had a large circle of friends and would go out to dinner, to the movies, or out for a drink with them—without Nancy. He often went to ball games or to watch sports on television with his male friends, and she felt slighted. She became frustrated and angry at Jay for having a social life separate from her, and felt that if she wasn't sexually available, maybe he would be more available to her. But the opposite happened. When she started to withhold sex it was obvious to him what she was doing, and that created more problems in their relationship. Eventually they split up. Nancy learned a valuable lesson, and although it cost her the relationship, she says she knows better for the next time.

Back in the 1950s it wasn't uncommon for a woman to believe that if she wanted a piece of jewelry from her husband, the way to get it was by having sex with him. Still, in a lot of relationships, women feel they have no power and sex is the tool they use to obtain some control, because ultimately the decision to have sex is the woman's. Her partner's needs and emotions are in her hands. And that's not a power that should be exploited.

The bottom line: Don't use sex to get what you want in your relationship. It will backfire.

KEEPING THE FLAMES BURNING

Passion is the glue to maintaining a strong, romantic relationship, no matter which phase of the relationship you are experiencing. Sexual contact is how men feel intimate and connected to their partners. It strengthens their emotional bond. Women, conversely, are sexually inspired when they feel emotionally close to their partners. So when sex and passion begin to disintegrate, the man will often feel less intimate, perhaps a little more withdrawn. In turn, the woman won't have the romance she craves in order to be sexually inspired and it becomes a vicious circle.

Sexual intimacy keeps the passion strong, but sometimes sex is more of a chore than a pleasure, especially after a full day of work, in or out of the home. So what can you do? Even if you are not in the mood, try to be intimate with your partner. Sometimes just hugging and kissing will do. Besides, once you get started you may change your tune.

Rekindling Passion: Jill's Story

Jill and Travis had been married for ten years and had two children under the age of five. Before the kids were born, they both thought their lovemaking was off the charts. Ever since they took their wedding vows, Travis was very romantic. He left tender little notes in Jill's purse at night, and she would find them while at work the next day. But with all the mounting responsibilities at home and work, sex was becoming less of a priority for Jill, and she became less sexually available to Travis. Those cute little notes became history. When she confronted him about his lack of interest and complained that he wasn't even giving her those tender bear hugs from behind when she was doing housework, he said it was because he felt disconnected. He blamed it on their absent sex life. She became incensed, accusing him of punishing her for not having the energy to make love. The tension heightened between them.

Laura worked with them, helping Jill realize that sex was the way Travis felt close to her and expressed intimacy, and it was that connection that inspired him to reach out romantically. They were at a stalemate and worked on ways to not only resume their sex life, but to make it better, even when she wasn't in the mood. Like so many couples, they had fallen into a rut. They simply went through the motions of sex, doing what they needed to reach orgasm, when emotionally they just weren't into it.

In therapy, they talked about various sexual positions they might try, different kinds of fantasies to explore. Jill admitted she was exhausted in the evenings, and Travis agreed to get up one morning every weekend with the kids so she could get some rest. Eventually things started to shift, and there was a change in Jill and Travis's sex life. He was making more of an effort in their relationship and she in the bedroom. They said it was an effort and took work, and they needed to mourn the loss of what their sex life was before they had kids, but they celebrated the life they had waiting ahead for them.

LOVE GAMES

Almost everyone who has kids finds it close to impossible to have a spontaneous sex life, and sex oftentimes has to be scheduled. Devising new ways to enhance your sex life is one way to reconnect. In *For Play: 150 Sex Games for Couples*, author Walter A. Shelburne, Ph.D., recommends 150 ways to spice up your sex life, making lovemaking more fun and exciting. Here are some games guaranteed to charge your sexual battery, including variations of Shelburne's *150 Sex Games*:

The wetter the better. Make love in the shower. Lather each other's body parts—and don't forget the erogenous zones!

Look Ma, no hands. Make mad passionate love with your arms behind your back. Instead, put your tongue and other body parts to use.

Naked chef. Cook together without any clothes on. See-through aprons allowed!

Strip Scrabble. Every time you score less than 15 points a word, you have to take off a piece of clothing.

Be a star. Take turns acting out different scenes of roles from sexy movies.

X-rated Twister. Play the game Twister naked.

Flash cards. Take turns drawing from cards that you and your partner have constructed. Each card has an intimate command written on it, with a word or phrase missing. Whoever pulls the card has to fill in the blank.

Scavenger hunt. Leave each other notes with instructions about what you must do to your partner when you find the item.

Truth or dare. Share your sexual fantasies with each other and invent an exciting way to fulfill them.

Just desserts. Have your partner close his (or her) eyes and scatter little pieces of fruit, candy, chocolate, and/or whipped cream all over his body. Then nibble them off.

Be prepared. Go on an outing to a secluded nature spot with a picnic lunch. Wear something easy to slip off. (You can even leave your underwear at home.) After you eat, make lovemaking your after-meal treat.

Go back to school. Buy a sexual technique manual at the bookstore or online. Then, with the book in your hand, climb into bed and practice anything new.

WHEN LOVE GOES AWRY: DEALING WITH INFIDELITY AND BETRAYAL

Regardless of how positive the relationship is, and even with marital vows, there can be trying times. Whether it's for love, sex, or to prove self-worth, both men and women are guilty of infidelity. Statistics show that one in five men and one in eight women have cheated on their spouse. Whether it's a one-night stand or a long-time affair, infidelity can spring from good marriages as well as unhappy ones. Still, whatever the reason may be, being the victim of betrayal is devastating. Typically, the scorned partner runs a gamut of emotions, including:

Denial. No matter how reliable the evidence, it may be hard to comprehend that you have been betrayed. But it's important to accept what has happened. Only then can you confront your spouse, deal with the issues, and move forward.

Self-blame. Believing an affair was your fault is not uncommon. But the truth is if there is discontentment in your relationship, your spouse should have dealt with any issues either by communicating his or her feelings, or through counseling, not by going outside of the relationship for sex. Sometimes the person who has strayed justifies an affair by claiming it was an unhappy union, when in fact that may not be the case at all. It is just a way to rationalize violating marriage vows.

> **87 percent of the women thought infidelity was always wrong.**

Rejection. Having your spouse cheat on you creates the ultimate feeling of rejection. It makes you feel worthless, unattractive, insecure, and lacking in sex appeal. But you have to realize it's your partner's difficulties and not your self-worth that is the problem.

Anger. It's a normal reaction to be furious when you learn your spouse has had an affair. But self-destructive behavior, such as blaming or devaluing yourself, won't accomplish anything. Don't allow the anger to consume you, destroy your self-esteem or appreciation of yourself, or spoil life's enjoyments.

If both parties are willing to salvage the marriage or relationship following an affair, forgiving and moving forward can be achieved. Many experts agree that infidelity can be a forgivable sin if the couple seeks help and confronts the different issues that may have instigated the betrayal. There are several steps involved in healing:

Don't expect a quick fix.

What to do: The affair has impacted on the basic fundamentals of your commitment to one another; the sense of trust, safety, and even familiarity has been broken. It takes a lot of work to move beyond an affair, and couples need to be prepared for a long haul. We encourage couples to commit to therapy on a month-by-month basis. At the end of each month they can evaluate their status, determine what has improved in their lives and their relationship, what healing has occurred, and what goals to set for the next month. This makes the healing process much more manageable.

Put it in writing.

What to do: Make an adultery contract where the adulterer promises not to cheat again and to cut off all communication with the other person. Unless he or she is willing to do so, it is impossible to move toward regaining trust. Part of rebuilding trust involves the adulterer keeping his (or her) partner informed as to his (or her) whereabouts. This reassures the betrayed party that nothing suspicious is taking place. To increase the trust in the relationship, the adulterer also needs to report back if the other woman (or man) has tried to make contact.

Get it out.

What to do: Vent the anger in a controlled way. The scorned spouse is often plagued with thoughts of the affair, many times even more so than the cheating partner. Typically, he or she will obsess about the times their spouse lied and the details of the betrayal. These thoughts are often accompanied by feelings of depression, lack of self-worth, and extreme anger. It is helpful for the one who has been betrayed to vent the anger in a time-limited way. This is also important for the adulterer. While there may be some self-loathing over his or her indis-cretions, it is hard to feel invested in the marriage when being con-stantly bashed for past behavior. We often advise couples to allow ten minutes a day for venting. The shattered spouse can yell, stamp, and scream, but only for ten minutes and then must stop. The one be-trayed should also be able to ask questions in order to move on, and the cheating partner must answer them. However, divulging gory de-tails of the affair should be avoided. It won't accomplish a thing.

Look Within

Look at yourselves as individuals. When Laura works with couples af-ter an affair, she finds that oftentimes the infidelity was not just about seeking sex. It's common for the spouse who violated the marriage vows not to feel any remorse, and it's common for the betrayed not to feel it was in any way her (or his) fault. Consequently, neither partner wants to accept responsibility. But in order for healing to begin, each partner—even the scorned—needs to explore personal issues that may have inspired the infidelity.

Sometimes it is low self-esteem or a symptom of a larger midlife crisis where the adulterer is questioning everything in his or her life, including work, marriage, and place in the community. Sometimes there is a family history of infidelity where having an affair was a "learned behavior" and condoned or encouraged. Did the victimized spouse suspect the affair was going on? What about their sexual needs, self-esteem, or family history? When something is happening in a relationship, it is rarely just one person's fault. Once there is clarity about what issues made either party susceptible to the affair, you can start working on yourselves and the relationship.

Reassess.

What to do: Look at your relationship. What was going on during the marriage? How was the communication? How active was the sex life? Infidelity is commonly a clue that something was amiss. It may be that marital conflict was the triggering event for one or both spouses to stray. When a couple is in therapy together, they can start to unravel the causes of the problems in the relationship and start the healing. The goal of therapy is to help the couple set up effective ways of communicating their feelings to one another, and help them come up with solutions for their conflicts.

It is a hard process to move through, both individually and as a couple, but it never ceases to amaze us how marriages can actually thrive after infidelity, sometimes better than before. An affair is a life-changing event for both partners, but once they do the work on themselves and their relationship, the marriage can be stronger than ever. So if you have been betrayed, don't throw out your wedding ring too soon. Your marriage may still be salvageable.

ASSURING RELATIONSHIP SATISFACTION

It's pretty much a given that we all want security and contentment in a relationship. But what are the components of a "satisfied" relationship? To begin with, it's a sense of safety and security, commitment, emotional support, tolerance, hope for a future. It's someone who loves you for you, including your faults. It's when you share trials, tribulations, joys, and accomplishments with your partner. It's also when you have a good sex life. Studies have shown that married women have better sex than unmarried women, probably because they feel safer and the commitment makes for a secure environment to explore their sexuality.

Have Your Own Interests

One of the predictors of a successful relationship, as discussed earlier, is when both parties have their own set of interests, friends, and sense of self, separate from their partner. When neither partner has an outside interest, the relationship can become suffocating and isolating. Although having something in common can add to a relationship, it is also important to develop hobbies of your own. It's when you become too wrapped up in your loved one, and too dependent on him or her, that you can lose your own identity, and the partnership will suffer.

Relationship Satisfaction outside the Bedroom

To be fully satisfied in a relationship, the majority of us need sexual intimacy. Sure, good sex is an aspect of relationship satisfaction, but it's not the only one. The totality of commitment enhances the physical connection, and for many, it's the intimacy that takes the relationship up a notch.

Relationship Satisfaction inside the Bedroom

Still, when sex isn't working, it becomes the key component in relationship dissatisfaction. When a couple's life is suffering from a lack of intimacy, either party can lose motivation to be sexual. Then, when the sex life starts to disintegrate, the following events typically start to happen:

The emotional intimacy breaks down. Men achieve emotional intimacy through sex. The more sex a man is having, the more romantically inspired he is. If sex isn't happening, he feels less close to his partner, and in turn, becomes less available. Eventually their emotional bond to one another and connection will break down.

There is a lack of affection. Physical affection stops. Gentle hand-holding, pleasing hugs, comforting caressing, and satisfying stroking can all start to disappear when sex in a relationship becomes nonexistent. That's because the partner who still wants sex doesn't want to reach out for fear of being rejected, and the partner who is avoiding sex is afraid that a little affection will be interpreted as an invitation for action in the bedroom.

There is a lack of connection. The couple starts to feel like roommates and becomes disconnected from the relationship. They may be great coparents or living partners together, but they might as well be just good friends. The "specialness" has left the relationship.

The emotional safety in the relationship dwindles. When sex isn't happening, the relationship can become more tense. The threshold at which they become annoyed with one another is lower, the ability to resolve conflicts is not as high, fights tend to come quicker and last longer. They don't have a basis of intense intimacy to keep them feeling safe with each other.

The question to ask oneself is whether your relationship is worth saving and/or at what point should you walk away? Everyone has different thresholds of what they will tolerate. It is usually not a good idea to walk away without trying to salvage the differences or exploring the difficulties, unless there is an abusive situation or a total lack of motivation by one or both partners to do the work to reconnect. If there wasn't an emotional or physical "connection" in the first place, the prognosis isn't good. But when both partners decide they want to be in the relationship and want to make it work, it's fixable.

BOTTOM LINE: DON'T DESPAIR

It can happen, desire can dwindle. Men and women, married couples in particular, have begun to speak out about their dwindling sex lives. In fact, the SWAN study (the National Institutes of Health's Study of Women's Health Across the Nation, an ongoing study reported on in the *Journal of Sex Research*) found that about 40 percent of women ages forty-two to fifty-two reported a low frequency of sexual desire. Even within a secure, solid marriage, some people are putting sex at the bottom of their list of marital priorities.

Whether it's due to a shift in hormone levels as women age, physical ailments, depression, side effects of medications, floundering economy, stress in the workplace, being consumed with the kids' activities, or just plain exhaustion at the end of the day, the end result can be problematic. And men, too, can experience a low sex drive for the same physical or emotional reasons as women.

The good news is a healthy sex life can be rejuvenated. If sex isn't your top priority, it doesn't mean you can't become aroused and enjoy it. For many people, once they engage in foreplay, arousal will follow naturally. For some, in order to get in the mood, they need to unwind. David Schnarch, in his book *Passionate Marriage*, suggests hugging until you relax and focus on your sensations. He says, "Once you've learned to make deep contact through it, you can extend the connection to intercourse."

Self-stimulation

Self-pleasuring, or masturbation, is a common practice among men and women alike, yet there is an embarrassment surrounding it. There shouldn't be. It can help a woman learn how to satisfy herself and share what feels good with her partner. In this chapter we focus on the benefits of self-stimulation and the techniques for going solo. It is one of the keys to great sex.

FINDINGS FROM THE WOMEN'S SEXUAL SATISFACTION SURVEY

- Sexually satisfied women place more importance on sexual satisfaction and being satisfied.
- Women who reported that they masturbated frequently were more satisfied sexually.
- Women who never masturbate placed less importance on sexual satisfaction.

Meeting Yourself for the First Time: Vanessa's Story

Vanessa grew up not knowing much about her body. The only time she even thought about her female anatomy was when she had her period. She never touched or looked at her genitals, and when she took a shower or bath, she would use only a washcloth, never her bare hands. This is what she had been taught as a child. She became sexually active when she was in her mid-twenties, but had a hard time becoming aroused and reaching an orgasm. When she turned thirty-two she came to see us for her low libido.

After Jennifer confirmed that there were no medical and/or hormonal components involved, Laura started to work with Vanessa to address the fact that she had no awareness of sensations in her genital area and had never experimented with self-stimulation. The first step in Vanessa's therapy was to familiarize her with her vulva, vagina, clitoris, and all other parts of her genitalia. The next course of action was to present the idea of self-stimulation. Vanessa began exploring her body, but before she could become comfortable touching herself, she had to work through the values that had inadvertently been passed down from her parents. She had to sort out what she had automatically internalized, and identify negative messages that affected her life. That took some effort, not to mention time, but it freed her up to the point where she was finally at ease touching her body.

Eventually she was able to reach orgasm through self-stimulation. She began using lubricants and vibrators and incorporated everything into her relationship with her partner. Masturbation allowed her to make a connection with her genitals in a way she hadn't before, and also played a healthy role in getting her on track sexually, alone and with a partner.

> **51 percent said they masturbate, whether it was rarely, sometimes, or often.**

THE M WORD

When Joycelyn Elders was surgeon general back in 1994, she made a statement that shocked many Americans. She suggested that masturbation should be taught in the schools. She paid a hefty price for that remark; it cost Elders her job, but it got people talking. A proponent of the dreaded M word, Elders believed that masturbation could help in the fight against HIV, theorizing that if young adults could self-stimulate, they wouldn't sleep around and put themselves at risk.

Whether that would hold true or not, we strongly agree that masturbation is perfectly normal. Defined as a sexual activity involving only one person, masturbation, or self-pleasuring, begins naturally at a very young age. From infancy little boys and girls touch their genitals because it feels good. They begin exploring their bodies and find the sensation of touching their genitals gratifying. It may start off to be unconscious, but by the time children are preschool age they are aware of the connection between touch and pleasurable sensations. Many children use it as a self-soothing mechanism and absentmindedly stroke themselves just because it makes them feel good.

Unfortunately, there has long been a taboo associated with masturbation. It was once considered the cause of all kinds of maladies, from mental illness to hairy palms to blindness. Even today, some religious groups believe that self-stimulation is a sin and a way of impeding conception, and that sexual pleasure should always be mutual, not to mention within the confines of marriage. In *A Celebration of Sex*, author Dr. Douglas Rosenau, a Christian sex therapist, writes that masturbation detracts from intimacy in marriage since it excludes the spouse.

For the most part, children learn to masturbate by self-exploration and trial and error even though they carry secrecy and shame. But self-stimulation is nothing to be ashamed of, and is a normal part of sexual development, not to mention an overall healthy sex life.

There is a school of thought, expressed by Elders, that if children were taught that masturbation was acceptable behavior and nothing to be ashamed of, they would make wiser sexual decisions. Self-stimulation would be an outlet for their sexual energy. What often happens with young people is that they have strong sexual urges but no idea what to do with them, and consequently they act impulsively. But if they could dispel that sexual energy in a safe way, it might prevent early sexual activity with random or casual partners.

THE ABCs FOR SELF-PLEASURING

How do you prepare? Firstly, ambience is everything. Create a calm, peaceful atmosphere by making sure you have some private, quiet space. Pour yourself a glass of wine, take a warm bath, turn on some soothing music—do what you have to in order to relax. Consider setting aside some lubricants. You can buy them at the drugstore or, even better, from erotica shops online, which often have a big selection.

To get started, here are some homework exercises that we suggest:

- **Look at anatomical drawings of the female genitalia to get a sense of where all the crucial parts are.**
- **Look at your own genitals in the mirror and identify all the parts.**

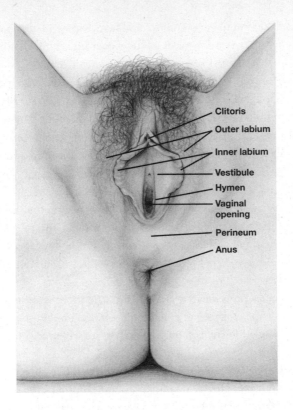

- **With your fingers and hands, touch all parts of your body.**
  Zero in on your erogenous zones. Stroke your breasts, shoul-
  ders, arms, stomach, inner thighs. Discover touching what body
  part sends chills down your spine.

For those of you who need a little more detail, here are some techniques we learned from sexually satisfied women:

Practice touching your genitals. Try rubbing different parts of your
genitalia—the labia majora, labia minora, urethra, clitoris, intervaginal
area, and perineum. The entrance to the vagina, the first third of the

vagina, is richest in nerve endings and many women like to touch themselves there. The goal is to get to know your body and what feels good.

Use different kinds of touch. Experiment with moving up and down, back and forth, or round and round. Try different frequencies of pressure—harder, softer, quicker, slower, faster. Some women find that if they stay in one area too long it starts to lose intensity. You can draw out and intensify the orgasm if you use the stop-and-start technique. When you feel yourself getting close to orgasm, pause for a second and then start again.

You may want to use one finger, two fingers, or more. Some women like to rub the larger area around the clitoris, some may like vaginal stimulation, and some prefer a combination of both. Try tightening and loosening your pelvic floor muscles while stimulating yourself.

Avoid making orgasm the goal. Just concentrate on arousal in the beginning. It may take some practice to self-stimulate to the point of orgasm. If something feels good, stay with it. It's a matter of trial and error.

Introduce vibrators. Go online or to an erotica shop and buy a vibrator. They can provide a kind of stimulation that human touch cannot. Orgasm can also be achieved easier with a vibrator.

Beautify the externals. Trim your pubic hair to give a heightened awareness, suggests Betty Dodson, a prominent sexologist who teaches women how to self-stimulate. She also recommends massaging the entire genital area with oils, generously applying lubricants, breathing fully when close to orgasm, searching your mind for erotic images, and experimenting with different bodily rhythms.

Of the respondents who reported masturbating often or sometimes, 41 percent masturbated alone only, 7 percent masturbated only with their partner, and 52 percent reported having done both within the past year.

GOING SOLO

Self-stimulating doesn't mean you are no longer interested in sex with your partner. In fact, it's just the opposite for some women—they say that once they become self-stimulators, they feel more erotic and more open to having hot sex with their partner. But that's not all. Women who masturbate reach orgasm easier. Those who expect their lover to deliver them to sexual ecstasy are oftentimes sorely disappointed. Unless you know from personal experience what kinds of stimulation you need, it's hard to give direction. You are the best judge of what arouses you. And keep in mind it's not cheating on your partner; rather, it's an opportunity to satisfy yourself without relying on another person.

> **28 percent felt it's easier to have an orgasm by themselves than with a partner.**

Believe it or not, self-stimulation has plenty of perks other than simply being pleasurable. Here are some of the benefits of solo sex:

- **IT HELPS YOU BECOME MORE SELF-AWARE. Women tend to have a disconnect between their genitals and the rest of their body, and usually think about them only during menstruation or when it's time for their annual gynecology appointment. But when you are connected to your genitals with regular masturbation, it can keep that mind-and-body connection going.**
- **IT CAN BE A LEARNING EXPERIENCE. It allows you to learn about your body. It helps to determine what is most sexually enjoyable for you, as well as how and where to be touched. As we age, our sexual needs change and regular self-stimulation can keep you attuned to what's presently satisfying. When you discover what you find most pleasurable, you can show your partner.**

- **IT KEEPS YOU TUNED IN TO YOUR BODY.** Self-stimulating is a way to keep tabs on your genitals. If anything changes or medical problems develop, you will be able to recognize any abnormalities.

- **IT HELPS KEEP THINGS DOWN THERE ALIVE.** When you masturbate you are keeping the pelvic-floor muscles toned and maintaining and stimulating blood flow to the area. It supports the "use it or lose it" philosophy. When there is the absence of a partner for an extended period of time, atrophy can occur. (There is no set time when atrophy sets in—it varies from woman to woman. The good news is that it can usually be reversed with the use of hormone replacement or vaginal hormone tablets.)

- **IT OFFERS SEXUAL RELEASE.** For women who are separated from their partners or husbands, or who are single and without a partner, it is a way to achieve sexual satisfaction alone.

- **IT ALLOWS FOR SEXUAL SATISFACTION ANY TIME.** No boyfriend? No problem. There is no waiting for a lover to engage in sex.

- **IT HAS CARDIOVASCULAR BENEFITS.** It's a good form of exercise. Your heart rate increases and your sympathetic nervous system goes into high gear.

- **IT CREATES RELAXATION.** It is conducive for sleep. Insomniacs will find masturbation can be as effective as a sleeping pill.

- **IT TAKES THE PRESSURE OFF YOUR PARTNER.** You can always rely on yourself to have an orgasm if your partner can't satisfy you.

TEAM APPROACH

Self-pleasuring in front of a partner can be embarrassing and daunting, but it is an opportunity to show your partner your sexually powerful sites. If your partner decides to join in, it's even better. Mutual masturbation can be a great turn-on.

There is nothing wrong with being the one to introduce mutual stimulation into the relationship, although it can be downright awkward. Many women worry that their partner may think they are kinky, and feel self-conscious or sheepish about doing something that has always been so private in front of someone. But just as your partner can see what sexually floats your boat, you can see what rocks his.

Yes, there are emotional risks, and yes, it means putting yourself out there, but it can be a bonding, erotic experience. For many, it's more intimate than intercourse, because it involves being more exposed. At first, masturbating in front of your partner may make it harder to reach orgasm because of the self-consciousness factor, but once a trust is built and there is an established comfort level it can be a major turn-on.

Bringing up the idea can be handled discreetly or openly. Here are some techniques that sexually satisfied women have shared with us:

Just do it. Begin self-stimulating in the middle of a sexual situation. Your partner will likely pull back and watch. If you want your partner to join in, say something like "Let me see how you touch yourself" or "Show me how you turn yourself on."

Make him guess. Build up anticipation. E-mail your partner or give a hint that you want to try something new that night. If your partner doesn't like surprises, you can tell him ahead of time. But if a man is interested in being sexual with you, he will most likely be receptive to the idea.

Fantasies and Erotica: Bonnie's Story

Bonnie, forty-four years old, had always been able to reach orgasm through self-stimulation and with a partner, but over the past few years she was finding she needed more stimulation in order to become aroused. Searching for a resolution, she started to explore fantasy, hoping that would enhance her arousal. At first, she read other women's fantasies, including *My Secret Garden* by

Nancy Friday. Reading other people's fantasies, she hoped, would act as a sexual inspiration. And it did. She wound up combining other people's fantasies with her own while self-stimulating, and that got her all fired up. It wasn't long before she started to create her own fantasies and her orgasms became more intense.

While some women rely on visual stimulation, such as watching videos, some read erotic books and others write their own make-believe scenario. Sexual fantasies are not only normal, everyone has them. Whether they are within the realm of reality or something totally off limits, they make arousal and orgasm easier.

These are some of the sexual fantasies reported by sexually satisfied women:

- **A hot and heavy sexual encounter with a present or past partner.**
- **Sexual submission—either they are being dragged away or are under someone's power.**
- **Sexual domination—they have control over their lover.**
- **Lovemaking with the same sex—they are having sizzling sex with another woman.**
- **Exhibitionism—an entire audience is watching them engage in spicy sex.**
- **Group sex—participating in a hot and heavy ménage à trois.**
- **Sex with a stranger—who is that masked man under the covers?**
- **Sex with someone they know other than their partner—anyone, from the hunk in the movies to that hot, cute guy at the health club.**

Anything goes with fantasies. That's what can make them so pleasurable. It's perfectly fine to let your mind wander. You can fantasize while engaging in self-stimulation and/or when having sex with a partner. Since this is your private, sexual magical world of make-believe, it's your choice if you want to share your fantasies or not. There is no right or wrong. Remember, the reason a fantasy is so powerful is because it's just that, a fantasy. It's not necessarily anything you would ever want to do in real life. Here are the cons and pros of sharing your secret sexual daydreams:

The Cons. It could be something so outlandish and far removed from anything realistic that you might be embarrassed or fearful it would be misinterpreted by your partner. Or it might be about someone you know, like a neighbor or even your partner's best friend, and sharing it might create relationship conflict or jealousy.

The Pros. You may have a storyline fantasy about being seduced or picked up that you can act out with your partner. If so, and you think your partner would enjoy or be receptive to playing it out, then sharing it will be fun. While you need to use your judgment, don't avoid sharing your thoughts because you fear that your partner might be shocked. Embarrassment shouldn't be an excuse. Your sexual wishes can be acted out, but ultimately the choice is yours.

> 11 percent of the respondents have bought vibrators or dildos within the past year. (The number in the survey was lower than we find in our practices. Perhaps it's because many women who use a vibrator got it from their partner or as a gift.) Of those women who masturbate often or sometimes, 37 percent reported using a vibrator.

GOOD VIBRATIONS

If you think that going out and buying a vibrator is inconceivable, think again. Sex toys are fast becoming common tools of self-stimulation, and respectable women, mothers, housewives, executives, teachers, lawyers, and physicians are among those who tread into that market. What's more, ways to buy them have gone beyond the local sex shop. Now slumber parties, or pleasure fairs, as they are sometimes called, are popping up all across America. The twenty-first-century hostess is not showing off samples of Tupperware, she is bringing in erotic gadgets and sex toys to demonstrate and sell. The support of other women, along with the sense of normalcy the parties provide, helps women muster up the courage to start exploring devices.

Therefore, if your orgasm or love life needs a little extra jolt, as in battery-operated or electric, think sex-cessory, think vibrator. It can heat things up in the bedroom, is a useful tool for a healthy sex life, and can help you learn what pleases you sexually.

The vibrator is not a new device. It dates back to the 1880s, says author Rebecca Chalker in *The Clitoral Truth*. She writes that they were even advertised in the Sears and Roebuck catalog, in which it was called a sexual health aid. Physicians and midwives believed that using a vibrator to stimulate a woman to orgasm was a way to deal with "hysteria."

It seems they vanished from advertisements after the 1930s, but resurfaced in the 1960s when women began to take notice of their "sexual benefits." Today many sex therapists endorse and advocate their usage.

With dozens of makes and models to choose from, vibrators come in a variety of shapes and sizes. They are made of rubber, plastic, or silicone and can be used for internal or external stimulation.

There are many common vibrator myths that may prevent you from partaking in this new arena of sexual exploration, and we're here to dispel those myths for you.

MYTH: If you masturbate you are no longer a virgin.
FACT: Only sexual intercourse can cause someone to lose their virginity.

MYTH: Masturbation can be injurious to your genitals.
FACT: There is nothing dangerous about self-stimulating unless you insert foreign objects into your vagina or urethra.

MYTH: Using your vibrator can become habit-forming.

FACT: You can always stop. Continue nonvibratory stimulation, either by yourself or with a partner. That way you both will remain confident that you're not becoming vibrator dependent.

MYTH: Using a vibrator means there's something wrong with you.

FACT: This is not true. Many people with full and happy sex lives use vibrators. It's just that no one talks about it. There is nothing wrong with wanting or even needing a little extra stimulation. It's harder for women to become aroused and reach orgasm than it is for men, especially as we age and have babies.

MYTH: The vibrator might replace your lover.

FACT: While no human will ever be able to provide the same kind of mechanical high-speed stimulation your device does, there's no substitute for the intimacy and connection you share with another person. Also, nothing can replace the feeling of warm flesh. So all you partners out there, don't worry. Using a vibrator does not mean that you are inadequate as a lover. If you're truly confident, you will probably enjoy it along with her.

MYTH: Your partner would never understand.

FACT: Most men thoroughly enjoy learning what arouses their partner and would find using a stimulation device exciting, assuming it's presented in a nonthreatening way. First, learn how to use a vibrator on your own, so you're comfortable with it and understand how it works. Then teach your partner how to use it. Bring it in as an adjunct to your lovemaking so that the vibrator doesn't steal the show.

The key to vibrator success is remembering that all vibrators are not alike, and because one is more costly than another doesn't mean it's better. We suggest starting with a simple external one, and not be drawn into buying a complicated device with rotating pearls, vibrating rabbit ears, or twenty settings. Later on, after becoming accustomed to using one, explore an internal or G-spot vibrator.

Check out the favorites we've learned about from our sexually satisfied women (and check out the appendix for Internet sites that sell them):

- **ACUVIBE.** Great standard for both beginners and advanced users. For external use and intimate massage, it's heavy duty, sturdy, and can last forever. It's electrical, but detaches from the power source in the plug. It can be used on your partner or even as a back massager.

- **BLISS.** This is well designed and contoured for a woman's body. It's battery-operated, has multiple speeds, is made of silicone, and considered a personal massager.

- **HITACHI MAGIC WAND.** This external electric vibrator is for the beginner who wants to experiment with self-stimulation. It's easy to control the intensity, has a wide head, and comes with attachments. With two different speeds, it's good for women with sensation problems, especially after childbirth.

- **THE JACK RABBIT.** This one makes it easy to customize the type of orgasm. It has rotating pearls in the center that allows for external and internal pleasure. But it's not for the beginner. If it sounds familiar, does *Sex and the City* ring a bell?

- **NATURAL CONTOURS.** Great for beginners or advanced, it comes in three sizes: petite, superbe, and magnifique. Shaped for a woman's body, it curves when it glides. Battery-operated, this external vibrator has three speeds and delivers vibrations to the clitoris and vulva.

- **THE PLEASURE COMMANDER.** A bullet vibrator with different rhythms and speeds. No bigger than your pinky finger, it's designed to be used alone or with a partner. There are attachments designed to be placed on your partner's penis, doubling the pleasure.

- **POCKET ROCKET.** This battery-operated vibrator is small and good for being incorporated into lovemaking. It's powerful and easily fits between two people. It even comes in a waterproof version and travels well.

- **VIELLE.** This does not vibrate; rather, it's a kind of finger cuff the woman or her partner wears to enhance stimulation and make it easier and quicker to reach orgasm. It is designed for clitoral orgasm.

If you really want to get hot and bothered, consider vibrating panties—they can add a whole new dimension to your sex life. They even come equipped with a remote control. That's right, your partner can turn them on from afar, but beware, the remote works for more than the panties. With a little click not only will your panties start to vibrate, but the woman down the block sporting them will also get a little jolt!

SHOPPING DILEMMA

Yes, purchasing a vibrator can be uncomfortable. But every major city has an array of female-friendly erotica shops that are not seedy, with salespeople trained to make you feel at ease. Couples can go together. It can turn into a romantic outing, and exploring the merchandise together will give an idea of what's the most inspiring.

If going to a shop is just too intimidating, shopping online is an alternative. It's possible to find what you are looking for from the privacy of your own home and have it delivered to your door. Drugstore.com, for instance, is one of the largest purveyors of sexual aids in the nation. Keep in mind, though, that one size doesn't always fit all.

> Women who bought more sex toys and other sexual aids placed more importance on sexual satisfaction.

FOR THE BRAVE HEART

If you are ready to move ahead, there is a pleasure world out there beyond vibrators. They are sex toys, and they open up a whole new vista of exploration for women. Probably the most common sex toy, aside from a vibrator, is a dildo. A dildo, usually shaped like a penis, doesn't vibrate and is more lifelike. It's often associated with lesbian sex and used with a harness to strap on to simulate intercourse. But many women enjoy using them alone, with a vibrator, or within a heterosexual relationship.

What else is out there? Pleasure kits, massage oils, clitoral stimulators, nipple clamps, blindfolds, erotic games, and edible treats to enhance sexual pleasure. Some games and toys are made of chocolate and can satisfy more than one kind of appetite. Pillows, too, can take on a different meaning. There are soft, fluffy pillows in all shapes and sizes to assist in different sexual positions. Each pillow makes way for a different pleasure. (See the Appendix for websites for sex toy shopping on the Internet.)

BOTTOM LINE

Masturbation can help you begin to understand how your body responds sexually, how to have an orgasm, and how to determine what you need to be satisfied. It can also act as a sensual type of foreplay. So, forget the embarrassment, ignore the taboo, and dump the guilt; masturbation is one of the keys to sexual pleasure. And it's practiced by sexually satisfied women. Whether you are married or single, male or female, it doesn't make a difference—you can and should reap the benefits of self-pleasuring.

Berman Footnote

Self-stimulation is not just a prescription for pleasure, it can also play a role in diagnosing sexual dysfunction. A woman may have difficulty becoming aroused or reaching orgasm and believe she is abnormal. Women who do not masturbate assume they have a problem having an orgasm when oftentimes the M word is the answer.

FIVE

Arousal, Lubrication, and Orgasm

When most of us think of satisfying sex, we think orgasm. Therefore it's no surprise that it's a key element of sexual satisfaction—as are arousal and lubrication, other necessities in ultimate lovemaking. In this chapter we explore what happens when arousal doesn't occur, and how to increase sensation and combat vaginal dryness. And we reveal tips on pleasure positions and achieving the big O.

FINDINGS FROM THE WOMEN'S SEXUAL SATISFACTION SURVEY

Sexually satisfied women say that:

- Orgasms are important, but not a key factor in their sexual satisfaction.
- Foreplay with their partner is arousing.
- Genital sensation is important for sexual satisfaction.
- Lubrication is a key factor that correlates with sexual satisfaction.

Lost and Found—Getting Your Sex Life Back: Ruth's Story

Ruth, a mother of four, was married for thirty years and always prided herself on having an exciting sex life. Between her children and her job she was constantly on overdrive, but that never stopped her from having blockbuster sex with her husband. Becoming aroused and reaching an orgasm were never a problem. However, as she started to move through menopause her hormone levels declined and she became less interested in lovemaking. Her diminished sex life created marital strife and she started losing that special connection she had with her husband. They began bickering, spent little time alone together, and became less intimate.

Ruth tried to force herself to become stimulated, but it didn't work. Worried about her waning sex drive and shaky marriage, she came to us for help. After weighing the risks and benefits of hormone replacement therapy, she decided to go that route, and within a few months started to feel better. She planned some romantic getaways with her husband, with no interruptions from the kids or office, and her once healthy sexual desire gradually returned.

While arousal is a major—and important—component of sexual satisfaction, it can't be forced. Arousal, the emotional and physiological result of sexual stimulation, is an involuntary response triggered only after becoming sexually excited. And women often take longer to become aroused than men, but hold on much longer.

Arousal is one of the five stages in the sexual response cycle. From pre- to postorgasm, the sequence of events is as follows:

1. **DESIRE.** It's the physical attraction, getting turned on and craving to be sexual with your partner. This is driven not only by the presence of hormones like testosterone, but by the emotional state of mind and feelings about the relationship.

2. **AROUSAL.** This is the excitement stage with physical changes. The vagina and vulva become moist and the clitoris and labia swell and become engorged; there is a tingling, warm sensation in the genital areas, flushing of the chest, and increased heart rate.

3. **PLATEAU.** It takes place right before going over the edge of orgasm. Arousal remains constant for a moment, then peaks. Muscle tension and arousal mount.

4. **ORGASM.** This is the peak of sexual response. There is an intense release of the vaginal muscles that built up during plateau.

5. **RESOLUTION.** The refractory phase. The vagina and clitoris go back to their normal states. Breathing slows down, flushing and swelling subside, and everything goes back to an unaroused state. Women, unlike most men, are capable of multiple orgasms, and can avoid the refractory phase with practice.

---

20 percent of the sexually active women said their sex life was negatively affected by not being able to achieve orgasm.

GOING HAYWIRE

Kissing, hugging, fondling just doesn't do it. Neither does a warm bath, a candlelit room, or an erotic video. No matter what you try, being aroused just isn't in the cards. Why is it that nothing seems to work? It could be for one of the following reasons:

Hypoactive Sexual Desire Disorder (HSDD)

This is characterized by a continuous lack of thoughts, fantasies, and motivation to be sexual. The cause can be medical, the result of medications, hormonal insufficiencies, or emotional factors such as depression, anxiety, or relationship conflicts. There is also a subcategory of HSDD called sexual aversion disorder, which is an almost phobic avoidance of sexual contact. This often stems from a history of trauma or sexual or physical abuse.

What to do: The first line of action is to focus on the lack of desire. To begin with, rule out any medical reasons with your doctor or treat the problem, whether it is your hormone levels or a sexual dysfunction (see Chapter 7). Next, think about, and improve, your relationship: Are you communicating? Are you struggling with anger? Do you have hidden issues? Do you feel a disconnect from your partner? Is there a lack of intimacy between you? Get it out in the open. Work on the relationship. A sex therapist may be helpful and/or necessary.

Female Sexual Arousal Disorder (FSAD)

FSAD is the inability to experience arousal. Age is not a factor—this can happen to old and young alike. Women with arousal disorders are unable to produce genital lubrication, do not have genital swelling or nipple sensitivity, find intercourse painful due to dryness, and have decreased clitoral and labial sensation.

What to do: There can be a number of causes of diminished desire, including low testosterone levels, low estrogen levels, stress, vaginal dryness, and depression. Talk to your doctor about possible underlying causes and treatment. (See Chapter 7 about more physical causes.)

Lack of Physical Attraction

You can't jump-start your sexual response if your partner doesn't turn you on. Sex appeal is very personal. It's like the old adage: One woman's poison is another woman's meat. For some that special appeal is a sense of humor, for others it's a husky build, and for others it's blond hair and blue eyes.

What to do: If you are able to call someone your partner, there must have been an attraction in the first place. So ask yourself what has changed? Did he gain fifty pounds or lose interest in his appearance? Did a bad-tempered side of his personality surface? If it's something eating away at you, gently bring it up. It is likely to be fixed. You can't force yourself to be attracted to someone, but if you once had it, then it may be regained.

> 38 percent of women said their sex life was negatively affected due to a lack of interest in sex.

Anxiety

If you are anxious, concentrating on your sex life isn't going to be easy. Generalized anxiety often causes excessive worries in one's life, as well as irrational fears, making it difficult to enjoy sex and sometimes life in general. Then, for some, just the idea of having sex sets them into a panic. Anxiety over having sex can stem from: guilt about experiencing sexual pleasure, concern your partner could injure your body, fear of a loss of control or loss of your own identity.

What to do: Get to the root of your anxiety and go from there. What's causing your stress? Consider relaxation techniques, exercise, and imagery, such as picturing yourself sunning on a sandy beach. If that fails, therapy may be the most helpful.

Exhaustion

Whether you are sleep-deprived or on overload at work or home, if you are too tired for leisure time, you will be too tired for an intimate encounter.

What to do: Don't take on more responsibility than need be. Try to get a good night's sleep. Don't begin a new activity shortly before bedtime. Avoid caffeine and alcohol a few hours before slipping under the covers. (You can find more about sleep deprivation in Chapter 7.)

Relationship Conflict or Resentment

Having a raging argument with your partner? Harboring anger? These feelings can put a damper on your sex life. If something with your partner is bothering you, it's hard to get past it to enjoy sex. When you feel troubled about your relationship, you are not going to feel like heating things up in the bedroom, much less be willing to experience the vulnerability that comes with having an orgasm.

What to do: Resolve any conflicts outside of the bedroom. Get off your chest what's bothering you, but don't be confrontational. That never works. And try to see your partner's point of view, too.

Berman Footnote

Although becoming sexually aroused is more difficult if you haven't had sex in a long time, keeping the blood flowing to the genital area will help maintain the health of the genital tissue. It doesn't mean you need marathon intercourse sessions, but with no sexual stimulation and no consistent influx of blood to the genital area, it might be hard to get aroused. The vaginal and clitoral tissue also atrophy and become less elastic or stretchy and less able to become engorged.

The Well's Run Dry:
Penny's Story

Penny was forty-eight years old with two children when she began missing her period. A blood test measuring her FSH (follicle stimulating hormone, which stimulates production of eggs in the ovaries) showed that she was in menopause. Up until that time she enjoyed a carefree, active sex life with her husband. But those days of raging hormones and natural lubrication were a thing of the past. Intercourse was now painful; even when she was aroused she was dry and sex was a hardship. Penny was afraid to admit to her husband that she was in menopause and made excuse after excuse to avoid sex. The lack of lovemaking began to take a toll on their marriage and she eventually broke down and told her husband what was happening. Upon the recommendation of her gynecologist, she started using a hormone patch along with vaginal creams. Eventually she became lubricated enough during arousal to enjoy a steamy love life.

When a menopausal or postmenopausal woman is moaning from pain instead of pleasure during sex, the likely culprit is a lack of genital lubrication. (Genital lubrication is a fluid released from the walls of the vagina that occurs during arousal when there is increased blood flow to the area.) When the vagina is dry, the friction of intercourse and penile penetration becomes painful and can cause burning or lacerations.

Many women, like Penny, are self-conscious and embarrassed when they are dry, and worry about responding sexually. When their partner notices there is a lubrication problem, they become even more anxious, inhibiting the arousal process even further. They also worry about sharing the news with their partner for fear of rejection.

There are several possible chronic and temporary causes for vaginal dryness, including:

Menopause

When estrogen levels drop and a woman becomes menopausal, the walls of the vagina become thinner; there is loss of elasticity and a diminished capacity to produce lubrication.

What to do: When hormone levels are dropping, they can be replaced. Products like VagiFem can replenish hormones and are only minimally systemically absorbed. They are little tablets inserted into the vagina that attach to the wall and stay in for a week at a time. Hormone replacement therapy (HRT) is another option, although it has not been without controversy. Studies like the Women's Health Initiative have linked synthetic estrogen and progesterone to breast cancer, Alzheimer's, stroke, and more. But for some it may be the best solution. The risks and benefits need to be evaluated. Check with your doctor.

Cold Medications

Antihistamines and decongestants can dry out the mucous membranes, including those in the vaginal walls.

What to do: Look for alternative drugs that can stop your sniffles but not your genital lubrication. Consider immunosupportive herbal approaches such as Emergen-C from the local health food store; it might help your body kick the cold without having to dry it out.

Vaginal Infections

They can lead to discomfort and reduce lubrication. Yeast infections are common culprits.

What to do: Any sign of an infection—redness, soreness, painful intercourse, pain during urination, or anything out of the ordinary—needs to be checked out by a doctor. Most bacterial infections respond to antibiotics, and yeast infections are treated with antifungal creams.

Not Enough Foreplay

If a woman isn't sexually excited enough she may not be able to produce vaginal moisture, and some women may need more time and more stimulation to become aroused.

What to do: Tell your partner you want more fondling, stroking, caressing, touching, deep kissing—whatever it takes to get your juices going. But don't just sit back waiting for it to happen; initiate, tantalize, excite, target his erogenous zones, work your way down his body—he will take the cue, and if he doesn't it's time to get specific.

Pregnancy and Breastfeeding

Estrogen levels decrease during breastfeeding. The good news is that when the milk stops flowing, hormone levels go back to normal.

What to do: It basically comes down to waiting it out. Over-the-counter lubricants can help with the dryness, but things should get back to normal three to six months after you stop breastfeeding. If they don't, see your doctor and make sure your hormone levels are back to where they should be.

Berman Footnote

Don't forget, if you don't use it, you might lose it. Becoming lubricated is more difficult when you haven't had sex in a long time. It doesn't mean you need regular intercourse, but with no sexual stimulation and no consistent influx of blood to the genital area, it might be hard to get aroused.

Also, a vasodilator like Viagra or one of the other drugs like it (Cialis or Levitra) should be considered if you have low arousal, especially if your doctor thinks the problem may be caused by nerve damage, aging, lack of use, or hormonal deficiencies.

If you think it's just for men, think again. Vasodilators increase blood flow for women, too, and lubrication is a direct result of blood flow. But don't just take your partner's pills. See your doctor and find out if you can take such medication.

If you have low sexual arousal, decreased sensation, or trouble achieving orgasm, talk to your doctor about the following treatment options:

LUBRICANTS

Drugstores, erotica shops, and websites carry a range of vaginal lubricants. Before using any lubricant, however, test it to make sure you aren't allergic. Put a drop on your arm and wait twenty-four hours. If there is no inflammation, redness, rash, hives, or swelling, it's probably safe for you to use. Lubricants are glycerin-, oil-,

silicone-, or water-based. Oil-based lubricants are not safe with condom use—water-based is the best when using a condom. Here are
some of our recommendations:

Uberlube

Pjur

Women by Body Glide

Vitamin E

Vielle Lubricant

Liquid Silk

Astroglide

KY jelly

**(Glycerin-based lubricants feel similar to Vaseline, whereas the water-
based lubricants are more liquid.)**

Topical Hormones

Local or topical estrogen relieves symptoms of vaginal dryness, burning, and urinary frequency and urgency. Some menopausal women
who complain of vaginal irritation, pain, or dryness are relieved with
topical estrogen cream. A vaginal estradiol tablet is another option—it
delivers low-dose estrogen locally and may benefit breast cancer patients and other women who are unable to take oral estrogen or use a
skin patch.

Estrogen Alternative

There is a new synthetic hormone available in Europe called Ti-
bolone, which can reduce vaginal dryness. It is a synthetic steroid
with properties similar to the body's natural steroid hormones (estrogens, progestogens, and androgens), which naturally stimulate libido
and vaginal lubrication.

PDE-V Inhibitors: Sildenafil, Vardenafil, and Tadalafil

Sildenafil (Viagra) promotes smooth muscle relaxation and increases blood flow. Women with low-arousal but healthy physiological hormone levels are good candidates for sildenafil to increase vaginal lubrication and clitoral sensitivity. Vardenafil relaxes smooth muscle and increases genital blood flow just like sildenafil. Studies show that vardenafil begins to take effect more quickly and has fewer adverse effects involving eyesight, the cardiovascular system, or digestive system. Tadalafil (Cialis) differentiates itself from sildenafil and vardenafil by staying in the system for up to thirty-six hours, increasing the opportunity to maintain the spontaneity in your sex life. Though FDA-approved only for use in men, the drug is undergoing global phase II trials for use in women.

L-Arginine and Yohimbine

These are sexual enhancement supplements. L-Arginine is an amino acid and yohimbine is an alkaloid agent.

Trouble with the Big O:
Pam's Story

Pam was a forty-seven-year-old stay-at-home mom with three children, ages eleven, sixteen, and eighteen. For years she was multiorgasmic, but as she became perimenopausal she started feeling more exhausted and having a much harder time reaching an orgasm. But for her it wasn't a problem, since she found the emotional connection and passionate buildup almost as satisfying as the big O. But her husband didn't agree. He was more goal oriented and couldn't understand why having an orgasm wasn't her priority.

Pam and her husband entered into therapy because she didn't want to start faking just to stroke his ego, and he needed some guidance to see her perspective. Together they worked out an arrangement. She would let him know when she had the energy or inclination to spend forty-five minutes to an hour to reach an orgasm, and he would accept it when she just wanted to make it a night of foreplay and intimacy, nothing further. It worked for them.

While climaxing may be the ultimate sexual experience for some, it's often not the most important element of sexual satisfaction. This is what the women in our survey say. There are many other factors that predict what satisfies a woman: intimacy in the relationship, the connection, and the overall sexual response. Yes, it's nice when orgasm happens and it's something to work toward, but it isn't always the epitome of the sexual experience.

> **53 percent of the women are dissatisfied if they do not have an orgasm.**
>
> **41 percent say they are not dissatisfied if they don't have an orgasm.**

THE ABCs OF ORGASM

Maybe you have never had an orgasm, or maybe you are not sure whether you've had one or not. We know most women don't achieve one every time they have sex, if at all. So what is an orgasm and how does it work? An orgasm is an involuntary response at the peak of sexual arousal following intense stimulation. When a woman is sexually aroused there is an increase of blood flow to her genitals, which feels like a pressure or fullness in the pelvis. She also may notice a kind of twitching of the pubococcygeal or pc muscles. Shortly, lubrication occurs in the vagina from the increased blood flow. That extra blood flow causes the upper two-thirds of the vagina to swell, the uterus and cervix to expand, and the clitoris to enlarge.

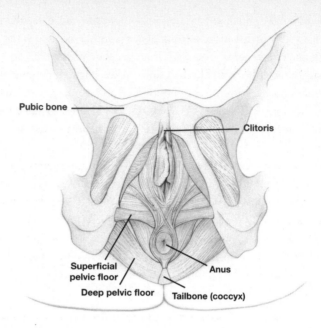

As a woman becomes more stimulated, her vagina becomes engorged with blood and swells along with the labia and clitoris. This swelling helps hold the penis. The inner lips, or labia minora, increase in size, pushing apart the outer lips and making vaginal penetration easier. Muscles throughout the body tense up, heart rate and respiration become rapid, and nipples may become erect. Ultimately an orgasm is an intense release of this muscle and pelvic-floor tension that feels pleasurable.

THE ROAD TO ORGASM

Having an orgasm isn't a matter of luck, it's knowing how and where to be touched and stimulated. Here are the ways to achieve supercharged orgasms:

Clitoral

This most common type of orgasm comes from continued stroking of the clitoris and surrounding area. The clitoris, which is comparable to the penis, is where the inner labia meet to form a hood at the top of the vulva.

Pelvic Floor or Vaginal

These occur by direct stimulation to that hidden treasure known as the G-spot, which creates a vaginal orgasm. The G-spot, first identified by German gynecologist Ernst Grafenberg in the 1940s, is a small mass of spongy tissue about the size of a small bean, located in the front wall of the vagina almost directly below the urethra—between the pubic bone and the cervix. The area swells when it's stimulated. This orgasm is reached by pressure on either the cervix or the anterior vaginal wall, or both. As we discussed in *For Women Only*, to find the G-spot, squat and explore the upper front wall of the vagina with your finger by applying firm, rhythmic pressure upward against the anterior vaginal wall. At first touch it feels like an urge to urinate, but that feeling passes. Women say this orgasm is oh so intense.

Blended

This one is a double header—it's a combination of the vaginal and clitoral orgasm. It can be reached by stimulating these erogenous zones at the same time. All of the areas can be massaged at once, or they can be alternated. Some say this is the ultimate pleasure.

PRACTICE MAKES PERFECT: TIPS ON REACHING AN ORGASM

While most women are capable of having an orgasm, many still have trouble achieving one. Even the most sexually active women experience obstacles. But if you have the desire and motivation, here is how to maximize your chance.

> **77 percent think it's easier to reach orgasm alone rather than with a partner.**
> **18 percent disagree.**

Tune in.
What to do: Pay attention to your physical sensations. Stay attuned to what's happening sexually with your body.

Tighten up.
What to do: Squeeze and release your pelvic-floor muscles repeatedly during stimulation, including intercourse (Kegel exercises).

Speak up.
What to do: You don't have to be a chatterbox in bed, but don't be shy, either. Ask your partner to stimulate you the way you like. Communicate what arouses you.

Get in the mood.
What to do: Get in a sexy mood beforehand. Take a bath, put on romantic lights, have a nice dinner, go dancing, do something you enjoy together.

Follow the golden rule.

What to do: Focus on your partner's pleasure, as you want him to pay attention to yours. This gives a sense of power, helps to lighten the mood, and takes the pressure off orgasm.

Fantasize.

What to do: Think of your fantasies during sex. Share them with your partner and have him share his. You can even act them out. Create new sexy scenarios together.

Keep eye contact.

What to do: Look in your partner's baby blues during sex. It heightens the connection and not only makes for a feeling of closeness but escalates excitement and decreases awareness of anything else but the moment.

Synchronize breathing.

What to do: Take deep breaths to relax.

Concentrate on pleasure.

What to do: Don't just think about your performance—or your partner's. Instead, savor the sensations and enjoyment.

Tune out the outside world.

What to do: Devote all of your attention to your sexual experience.

Pay attention to all the physical sensations.

What to do: Tune in to how the air feels on your skin when you first get undressed, to your partner's touch. Note your emotional sensations as well.

Imagine.

What to do: Think about a particular idea or image of melding with your partner, perhaps on the sensation of opening up to your partner or squeezing him during intercourse.

Speak up.

What to do: Talk or make sounds during sex: say your partner's name, "I love you," moan, tell your partner how good it feels, talk dirty. This all keeps you in the moment.

You don't have to twist or strain your body or be a contortionist to achieve out-of-this-world orgasms. Here are some tried-and-true positions for increasing a woman's sexual satisfaction:

The missionary position.

What to do: The basic missionary position can be unsatisfying for many women because it can be hard to achieve clitoral or G-spot stimulation. But with some simple variations, this old standard can increase your partner's ability to stimulate the clitoris and G-spot, thereby heightening your pleasure and helping you achieve orgasm. Lie on your back, under your partner, with your pelvis tilted upward. Your vulva should be angled so that it presses flat against your partner's pelvic bone and causes friction on the clitoris, urethra, and labia minora. Try placing one or more pillows under your hips and experimenting with different angles to see what works best and offers the best stimulation. For a variation and to allow for deeper penetration, you can wrap your legs around his waist or pull your knees up to your chest.

The standing position.

What to do: This position can provide simultaneous clitoral and G-spot stimulation. Stand facing each other while your partner leans against something behind him so that he is positioned slightly beneath you, then rock back and forth while he thrusts at an upward angle against your G-spot.

The Coital Alignment Technique (CAT).

What to do: This provides direct stimulation to the clitoris. Your partner should lie across your body without putting his weight on his elbows. He should shift his pelvis from the standard missionary position to line up his pelvis with yours so his penis makes direct contact with the clitoris. Engage in a rhythmic, back-and-forth rocking motion rather than penile thrusting. Move upward while your partner presses downward, making sure that the penile-clitoral connection is maintained through pressure and counterpressure.

Be on the top.

What to do: This lets the woman move her pelvis so that she controls the friction and position of the penis as it rubs against her labia and clitoris. With your partner either lying down or sitting up, engage in a rocking chair motion. This face-to-face position can allow for deep thrusting into the vagina, which can lead to stimulation of the cervix and a pelvic-floor or clitoral orgasm.

THE PLUSES OF ORGASM

While orgasm is not a critical element in a woman's sexual satisfaction, it's nice when it happens. If you have orgasmic success, you want more because it feels good. Here's what else it can do:

- **ALLEVIATE STRESS. Following an orgasm, the hormone dopamine is released and the body experiences a period of relaxation.**

- **CREATE FEELINGS OF BONDING.** The shared experience can make you feel closer to your partner.
- **REDUCE DEPRESSION.** It tends to release the endorphins, feel-good chemicals that enhance your mood.
- **ALLEVIATE MENSTRUAL CRAMPS.** The uterine contractions help to loosen up the muscles that are contracting around the uterus, causing the cramps.
- **PROVIDE GOOD EXERCISE.** It puts a lot of stress on the sympathetic and parasympathetic nervous system, which increases breathing and heart rate. The muscle contractions can be beneficial to blood flow as well as muscle tone.
- **INDUCE SLEEP.** Commonly, sleepiness occurs following orgasm.

COMMON MISTAKES

A lot of factors affect having an orgasm—ambience, sexual positions, state of mind, to name a few. But there are triggers that are bound to set the stage for an uneventful evening of lovemaking. Do any of these sound familiar? If so, take notice of how and how not to savor the experience:

MISTAKE: Bringing your worries to bed.
SOLUTION: Avoid distractions. When you are in the throes of passion, try to push the bad day at the office or your kid's report card out of your mind. Daytime worries are not conducive to an orgasmic evening.

MISTAKE: Rushing through.
SOLUTION: Don't hurry love. Maybe you have to get up early to take the kids to school, or set the alarm for an early-morning meeting, but for women, reaching an orgasm takes time. Enjoy the foreplay, take the time to cuddle, and concentrate on the passion.

MISTAKE: Focusing too much.

SOLUTION: Be in the moment and don't lose sight of the process. Instead, pay attention to sensations and the erotic feelings, the connection and what is happening in your body. Don't obsess about whether it's working, your partner's expectations, or if you are close to orgasm.

MISTAKE: Being embarrassed.

SOLUTION: Women who feel self-conscious might have difficulty reaching orgasm. But take a risk, let yourself go, and don't hide under the covers if you don't or can't.

MISTAKE: Taking your relationship conflicts into bed.

SOLUTION: It's hard to get aroused when you are confronting any problems in your relationship. Leave any personal strife outside of the bedroom.

BEYOND INTERCOURSE

It's not surprising how many women, married or not, have never had an orgasm. Paula was married for five years and had sex regularly with her husband, but never experienced orgasm. She said the steps were always in place. She was caressed, kissed, and massaged. Her vagina was lubricated, sexual tension heightened, and clitoris stimulated. But during intercourse, she never felt those waves of muscular contractions and spasms in her vaginal area followed by a terrific sense of relaxation.

Intercourse alone doesn't necessarily provide the intense stimulation needed to achieve orgasm. As mentioned in *For Women Only*, Laura calls nonintercourse sex VENIS—Very Erotic Non Insertive Sex. All couples, especially those in which one partner suffers from sexual dysfunction or severe vaginal dryness, can give each other sexual pleasure in ways that do not require penile penetration. Many gay women enjoy sex this way. It is foreplay to the max. It is an alternative to safer sex because there is no exchange of bodily fluids.

Possible erotic and sexually stimulating activities that may or may not lead to orgasm, include:

- **Erotic wrestling with maximum body and genital contact**
- **Massaging each other with oils or other materials**
- **Light bondage with fur or feathers**
- **Mutual masturbation**
- **Erotic dancing**
- **Intercourse between breasts or buttocks**
- **Body kissing**

Not all couples engage in VENIS because of an inability to reach an orgasm. Many incorporate VENIS as a variation from their regular sex life. VENIS requires verbal and nonverbal interaction between partners, which overall helps to improve sexual satisfaction and sexual communication skills.

TROUBLE ACHIEVING ORGASM

You may go through ebbs and flows in your ease and ability for reaching orgasm, depending on your body, your mood, and who you are with. But if the problem persists, it may be time to take a second look. Maybe you never had an orgasm, or you once could but are no longer able. Perhaps you have always been able to reach one with self-stimulation but not with a partner. Or possibly you have orgasms with a partner but never during intercourse.

Whatever the case, difficulties need to be addressed. Here are physical and emotional reasons why women can't reach orgasm:

Physical reasons. There are a number of physical reasons for why one can't reach an orgasm. See Chapter 7 for physical/medical or orgasmic dysfunctions as well as treatments.

Sexual trauma or abuse history. For anyone who has grown up amid abuse, it is bound to have a profound affect, sexually and otherwise. A history of sexual abuse can lead to inhibitions or difficulties with sexual desire, arousal, or pain disorders.

Depression. It lowers one's interest in sex and enjoyment in general. It causes withdrawal, irritability, sadness, a feeling of hopelessness, and the lack of a desire to do anything pleasurable.

ADHD (attention deficit hyperactivity disorder). Laura has found in her clinical practice that women with ADHD often have difficulty staying mentally present and focusing on their sexual arousal. Furthermore, many of the medications used to manage ADHD symptoms have sexual side effects as well.

Ashley's Story

Ashley was a thirty-two-year-old writer and married for three years. She came to Jennifer pleading for help, saying her marriage was over. Ashley has multiple sclerosis, and as a result, she struggled with a variety of symptoms, including the change in her ability to achieve orgasm. Jennifer's approach to Ashley's problem was twofold: to help her work through her marital-relationship issues and to focus on her physical problem. Ashley's MS was the root of her emotional problems, which affected her sex life, and therapy was recommended. Medically, Jennifer prescribed blood flow–enhancing products like Viagra and Levitra, and Ashley was able to reach orgasm.

Orgasmic disorder is one of the hardest sexual function complaints to treat, especially if it is a lifelong problem. Orgasm is a learned response that occurs at the time of puberty if not earlier. As one might assume, the market is ripe with potential treatments that claim they can deliver women to ecstasy with the push of a button, a magic injection, or a special pill. But beware, unless these interventions have clinical, placebo-controlled trials to back up their safety and efficacy, you should not be fooled. Here are a couple of the latest treatments that have gained a lot of attention in the media:

The Orgasmatron

This device is named after the one made famous in the Woody Allen movie *Sleeper*. Basically, the orgasmatron is a type of pacemaker. An electrode is implanted in the lower spine and attached to an electrical stimulator pack (about the size of a pack of cards) that is placed under the skin in the buttocks. Mild electrical pulses travel from the pack to the probe, stimulating the sacral nerve in the spine; patients can control the level of stimulation via a remote control. The orgasmatron was developed after women with similar implants, designed to manage chronic back pain or bladder control problems, reported that the device was giving them an orgasm. When that area of the spine was stimulated, genital stimulation was produced as well. This device is presently being studied in clinical trials as a potential treatment for orgasmic disorder.

Collagen

Another controversial new development in the search for the ideal orgasm is a new trend a few clinicians are advertising that involves the injecting of collagen in the G-spot. The idea is that the collagen enlarges the surface of this sensitive area, making it easier for a woman to be stimulated to orgasm. However, this procedure has not been tested for effectiveness or safety, and Kegel exercises and learning to use the muscles surrounding the vagina can provide as much stimulation to the G-spot as an injection.

FAKING AN ORGASM

Faking an orgasm is never a good idea. Not only does it break the trust in the relationship, it also puts too much emphasis on climaxing. Why would someone fake? For plenty of reasons: To take the focus off themselves and avoid the pressure of reaching an orgasm; to please their partner; to make the sexual act end quicker. Or to avoid discussing the reasons why they may not be having an orgasm. But communication is important, and when the partner finds out she lied, he may feel betrayed, disappointed, and hurt.

The problem with faking is that it eventually comes out, either by mistake or by design. Many women say they finally admitted it because they wanted to start working on reaching orgasm with their partner. The problem is that when she tells her partner she's been faking, they may start having sexual functioning problems as well. He (or she) starts to feel inadequate and unsafe, wondering why she felt the need to lie and what else she is keeping from him.

Keeping a Secret:
Jeanne's Story

Jeanne was in her late thirties and was never able to reach orgasm. Every time she was with a new partner she would tell him her dilemma and he would take it as his personal goal in life to be the one to bring her sexual bliss. Then she met Max, whom she wanted to marry. He, too, wanted to be the one to help her reach an orgasm, so she eventually started to fake it, to give him the validation that he wanted. They married and for several years she took the easy way out and continued to fake it. She was afraid to confess since so much of his pride was related to being the one to finally give her an orgasm.

Instead of telling him the truth, she decided to start working on her own self-stimulation and arousal, and eventually learned to reach orgasm alone. Once she accomplished that, she told Max she was finding it more difficult to respond and wanted to try some new techniques in their sex life together. He was open to her suggestions and was able to learn the stimulation techniques she introduced to him. Ultimately Jeanne was able to reach orgasm with him. He never knew that she went from faking it to the real thing.

Honesty Turned Out to Be the Best Policy: Kelly's Story

Of course, not everyone's story has a happy ending. Kelly, in her early forties and going through perimenopause, started to have sexual response problems based on the changes in her hormone levels and decreased genital blood flow. She confessed to her partner that she was having a difficult time reaching orgasm, but he took it personally, so she found it easier to pretend. After a while it started to affect her libido. She felt resentful of his ability to reach orgasm every time, and annoyed with how pleased he always seemed after she faked. Finally Kelly decided to tell her partner the truth, that she was not as responsive as she seemed and that her sexual response had changed. She suggested trying extra stimulation in order to reach orgasm. But instead of focusing on how to solve the problem, her partner couldn't get past the fact that she had been pretending. He became extremely upset and felt betrayed. They moved beyond it, but it took a lot of work and a long time for him to feel safe with her again.

In building trust in a relationship, it's important to discuss any difficulties with your partner. Understand that only about one-third of women reach orgasm with intercourse, and only half of women reach orgasm on a regular basis. You need to educate your partner. He may believe that in his experience all the women had an orgasm, but in truth those women may have been faking it, too.

For men more than women, reaching an orgasm is a motivating part of the sexual act. Men want to satisfy their partner, be the sexual hero, which is a big part of their sense of self-esteem, virility, and strength. It's a myth that men are selfish in bed. In general, when a man is invested in a relationship, he wants his sexual partner to enjoy the full experience.

EROGENOUS ZONES

When you hear the words *erogenous zones*, most likely genitals come to mind. But our sex organs aren't the only part of our body that can be sexually sensitive. Many other parts of a woman's, and a man's, body are rich in nerve endings, and massaging them can heighten sexual pleasure.

What are some of those personal secret spots? Inner thighs, back of the knees, back of the neck, behind the ears, lower back, feet and wrists, the buttocks, and nipples are all fairly common sensitive areas that when caressed can start your sexual engine.

Women seem to be more sensitive around their erogenous zones than men. We suggest to couples that they draw an outline of the woman's body and separately mark her erogenous zones in the order she typically likes them, then compare drawings. Then do the same with an outline of a man's body. You may be surprised; even couples who are married, or have been together for a long time, have very different perceptions. This is a way to discover something new and open the door to sexual communication between you and your partner.

When stroking sensitive zones, think beyond maneuvering with your hands. Think about your tongue, forearm, hair, fingers, or even feathers or silk—they can prove to be oh so titillating.

ALONE TIME

We can't complete this chapter without mentioning again the role of self-stimulation and orgasm. As we talked about in the last chapter, it's easier to reach orgasm alone than with a partner. You can control the stimulation without any pressure or expectations from another party. We recommend that women learn to have an orgasm alone first and then teach their partner what to do. When women leave their orgasm in the hands of their partner, it applies a lot of pressure and creates unrealistic expectations. That's why taking control of your own sexuality and learning about your own body is a key part of orgasmic health.

BOTTOM LINE

When it comes to sex, more is definitely better. Sexual arousal keeps your genitals alive and healthy and prevents them from aging. Although arousal is necessary for orgasm to occur, don't be hard on yourself if it doesn't happen every time. If you practice often and use the tools we mentioned in this chapter, you're sure to have one more often than not.

Addressing Your Past

Most of this book is focused on the positive aspects of our sex lives. It's loaded with tips, tools, and rules. However, we don't think we can do an effective job in laying out the foundations of sexual satisfaction without taking a look at the past. What goes wrong in a person's sexual development can play a role in preventing or reaching sexual satisfaction. Therefore, in this chapter we want you to explore experiences encountered during maturation. We find that sexually satisfied women face and address their past, and that's an essential component of enjoying a healthy and happy sexual life. How your caregivers or parents interacted sexually with each other, how they treated sex, how they reacted when you began menstruating, the

---

FINDINGS FROM THE WOMEN'S
SEXUAL SATISFACTION SURVEY

- Those who reported abuse and received counseling reported higher sexual satisfaction, compared to those who had been abused and didn't receive counseling.

---

impact of your religious training, your first sexual experience, are all part of your sexual development.

Instead of us telling you "how to," we have included pointed questions for you to ask yourself that will help you recall your past. You will track your own sexual history, explore your family dynamics, identify patterns, and see how they are expressed today. Is it easy? No. Is it fun? No. But it's a big piece of the puzzle and a crucial step in achieving sexual satisfaction. So get ready to walk down memory lane—for better or for worse.

Moving On:
Stacey's Story

Stacey, along with her three siblings, grew up in a home with abusive and neglectful parents. Not only did Stacey's mother and father call her hurtful names and slap her time and time again, but they would leave her and her siblings alone for days without any adult supervision. When Stacey was old enough to date, she made one poor choice after another. She felt worthless and undeserving of tender loving care. The males she picked were emotionally and physically abusive to her—just like her parents.

After two failed marriages, a very unhappy existence, and an unsatisfying sex life, Stacey felt she hit rock bottom and decided to seek therapy to change her path of self-destruction. It took several years of intense psychotherapy and self-exploration before she could understand her destructive behavior. Only then could she make positive changes in her life and move on. Stacey is now happily married with three children and a thoughtful and loving husband. Her sex life has gone from fairly unpleasant to very satisfying. Without dealing with her past, Stacey would not have been able to resolve sexual conflicts, overcome stumbling blocks, and move forward and enjoy sex.

RECORDING YOUR HISTORY

The first step in addressing your past is setting some time aside to carefully think about all your sexual experiences and influences. In recalling your sexual history, try writing everything down. Having it down on paper may make it easier to identify patterns and see where any difficulties originated. What kinds of issues may surface? Anything and everything, so leave no stone unturned. For example, if you never saw affection between your mother and father, write it down. And if you have difficulty giving and receiving affection, note that, too.

Getting Started

To help organize your memories, after each section we will present key questions for you to ask yourself. Try to recall not only the memories of the experiences, but the feelings you had at the time. For instance, if after the first time you had sex you felt giddy and happy that you gave yourself fully, jot it down. Or if after the first time you felt guilty, saddened that you lost your virginity, regretted it, couldn't concentrate in school, note that.

How can understanding your sexual history benefit you in the long run? Here's how:

Gets to the roots. It allows you to see the source of your problems and helps you to move forward. Becoming familiar with your sexual history, especially recognizing repeated behavior, enables you to leave the past in the past and be free to make healthier choices in the present.

Gives you insight. It allows you to look at your family dynamics around sexuality, and the messages you received growing up. It gives you a chance to look at your family values objectively. One of the biggest challenges for all of us in adulthood is to be able to separate our own values from our family's. We all carry the value systems we grew up with, which may not necessarily be beneficial as we get older. Having a chance to look back objectively at those values can either be validating, or can help you move away from them.

Gives you empowerment. Knowing your sexual history plays a role in your sexual empowerment—it's taking control of your sex life and facing any stumbling blocks. Growing up, our sexuality is strongly influenced by our parents and their values and prejudices, and what they believe to be acceptable or unacceptable. Your sexual development may have been distorted by fear or disappointment or guilt, and until you identify where those emotions originated, you can't become sexually empowered or satisfied. It's hard to be empowered if you haven't separated your feelings about sexuality from those of your parents.

Like Mother, Like Daughter:
Michelle's Story

Michelle, age thirty-seven, wasn't able to enjoy sex with any of her boyfriends, no matter what she did. She believed that men couldn't be trusted, and felt their only interest in women was for their own sexual gratification. Yet, she knew that her friends didn't feel the same way, and that her view of men was distorted. Wanting to change, she entered into therapy. The first step was to explore where this line of thinking came from, and she was able to trace it back to her mother. Michelle's parents had an unhappy marriage, and her father was unfaithful. Growing up, time after time, her mother complained to Michelle about men and sex. She admitted to Michelle that she hated it when her husband (Michelle's father) touched her. So when Michelle entered into adulthood, it was difficult for her to shake those negative messages. She had a hard time separating her own viewpoint from her mother's.

It took some work for Michelle to understand that the attitudes she developed were really her mother's and not her own. She came to realize that her mother was a product of her own environment, raised in a strict, conservative home with a father who made her feel guilty for even thinking about sex. Over time, Michelle recognized that she didn't have to take on the attitudes that were based on her mother's childhood wounds, and she started to feel better about her partner's advances. Her mind-set changed, and she began to allow herself to actually enjoy having sex.

As with Michelle, if your issues are deeply rooted, they may be resolved only with the help of a trained therapist. Writing your own sexual history can highlight areas that need to be worked on and provide your therapist with a road map of your sexual issues. If you enter therapy knowing the key elements that are holding you back, the treatment process will go much quicker.

DIGGING DEEP

In doing a sexual history, it is possible that memories will surface that have been repressed. When there is a trauma the incident may be buried or pushed aside, and a simple question may bring up the memory. However, many people with a traumatic sexual history will have an inkling that something bad took place, even if they don't consciously remember it. In some cases, it's too deeply buried to be brought out by a few questions. If you go through this process and remember an incident that you haven't thought about but that implies you had some sort of abuse or trauma, it is crucial to get professional help. Bringing up that pain again requires the help of someone trained to help you cope with and resolve it.

Be aware, however, that having been abused doesn't mean a life of doom and gloom. Sexually abused women can reach a resolution and go on to have a fulfilling love life. Depending on the trauma and how it was dealt with at the time, a woman can enjoy healthy relationships as an adult. With the help of a therapist, a sexually abused woman has to experience a series of stages before finding herself on the road to recovery. She has to:

- Acknowledge what happened
- Recognize it wasn't her fault
- Purge the humiliation and guilt
- Let go of the pain and redirect the anger at the perpetrator.

Be aware that each of these steps is a part of healing and can involve a process of personal exploration and guidance and therapy from a trained professional.

Learning About Sex:
Vicki's Story

When Vicki was eleven years old she overheard some kids on the playground saying the f word. She didn't know what it meant, and innocently asked her parents at the dinner table. Her father stood up and yelled at her never to use that word again, and asked her to leave the room. It was a humiliating incident that Vicki never forgot. From that moment on she never talked about sex with her parents. She got a clear message that sex was something bad, and certainly something never to be discussed. When she grew up, she vowed to always have open communication with her children and to welcome any questions.

Vicki's experience is not unique. Many parents avoid the "birds and the bees" discussion because they are uncomfortable or embarrassed. Although ideally parents should be the ones to teach their children about their bodies, genitals, reproduction, and sexuality, oftentimes that doesn't happen. When we ask patients where they got their sex education, many say from friends, less than half say from their parents. In fact, many feel uneasy discussing sex at all with their mother and father. But when youngsters get their sex education from their peers, it's likely they did not get all the facts. Parents are much better equipped to give accurate information and provide a healthy attitude about sex, without being too explicit.

Shondra's Story

When Laura was in graduate school working at a teen AIDS/HIV testing center, she counseled Shondra, a very anxious and shaken-up fourteen-year-old girl who came to the center for AIDS testing. She had come from a very restrictive family background and never received any sex education. Her family refused to let her take health education in school simply because they talked about sex in the class. Because of her naïveté she was faced with a sexual situation she did not know how to handle. She didn't know what sex was, let alone safe sex, and found herself at a party with a high school student trying to have intercourse with her. Although she consented, it was basically rape because she didn't know what was going on or how to stop it. She didn't have the ability to say no. She had no preparation, no precautions, no condom or any awareness of what condoms are used for. Luckily she was disease-free and she wasn't pregnant, but she was terribly ashamed and guilty and that experience was clearly going to set the tone for the rest of her sexual life.

For sure, being armed with information about abstinence and protection gives you the confidence to say no, or negotiate for safer sex. But if you were like Shondra, naive and uninformed, and were pressured into having sex against your will, the experience could have been emotionally damaging.

QUESTIONS

- Did your parents tell you about sex and how babies were born? If so, how?
- How did they react when you raised questions?
- Did they call the genitals by their proper names?
- Did they discuss intimacy and sex openly in the house?
- Did your parents talk to you about sexual abuse, AIDS, pregnancy, rape, and/or sexually transmitted diseases?
- What kind of impression did they give you about sex?
- How did your parents handle sexual boundaries?
- Did they give you privacy and did they allow you to lock your door?
- Did your parents accuse you of being sexual even when you weren't?

TOUCHY FEELY

When examining your family history, think about the physical messages you received early on. The ideal is growing up in a home where your parents were affectionate toward each other and you. Hugging, kissing, cuddling lay the groundwork for sensuality, as sensory development is a key component of sensuality later in life. It doesn't mean that babies or children feel sexual when being touched or cuddled by their mother or father; rather, they are having the experience of closeness and intimacy and it feels good. Affection should be a part of a child's overall experience with people they love. When raised with affection, a child develops a sense of security, containment, and safety.

Often we see couples where one, or even both, has difficulty showing affection. They have a hard time holding hands or touching each other because they weren't raised in a family where affection was expressed openly. When you grow up with a lack of affection, you may have trouble giving or receiving affection later on.

Of course, there are nurturing mothers who adore their children but are psychologically unable to show physical affection. Perhaps they themselves were brought up in rigid homes where touching wasn't commonplace. Unless you had a modeling of what connection, intimacy, and affection are, it's hard to achieve that later in a relationship. If you never saw your parents cuddling, it's very hard to explore that area of your sensuality later because it doesn't come naturally to you. But the cycle can be broken.

Another avenue to explore is your parents' sexual relationship. You may have seen your father trying to hug or kiss or hold hands with your mother and she pulled away, or your mother reaching out to your father but he was unresponsive or unaffectionate in return. That coldness and rejection you witnessed can be passed on to you, especially if you didn't receive affection. You may be less likely to express affection for fear of a negative reaction, or you may feel ambivalent, untrusting of men, and uncomfortable reaching out for fear of being rejected yourself.

The emotional love and affection we get from our parents is imprinted on us in terms of how we feel about ourselves, and how we experience ourselves in the outside world. From the time we are babies, love and affection has an impact on our well-being. Kids need some degree of care and physical connection in order to be emotionally and socially healthy as they grow up.

During World War II there were several studies that showed the negative effect the absence of parents can have on children. In one such study, Dorothy Burlingham and Anna Freud found that the children who were evacuated from London and separated from their mothers had behavioral difficulties.

Other studies, too, showed that children in hospitals and institutions, who were separated from their mothers, even if it was for a brief period, were found to have psychological disturbances.

A recent volunteer program at St. Luke's–Roosevelt Hospital Center in New York City looked at infants who were abandoned, neglected, or born drug-addicted or with AIDS. Although they were given good medical care, they received no nurturing. They stayed listless and didn't even react to sound. But when volunteers held and rubbed the babies they became alert, smiled, and cooed.

If you didn't receive any affection from your parents, you may be uneasy with that kind of expression, and your sense of self-worth and ability to give affection with comfort may be compromised. We often emulate our parents once we find ourselves in similar roles, without even realizing it. If this sounds familiar, know that, depending on the degree of affection and neglect, it can be overcome with awareness and hard work.

QUESTIONS

- Did your parents hug and kiss you when you were growing up?
- Did you feel comfortable cuddling with your mother and father?
- Were you ever rejected when you tried to express affection?
- Did you feel secure in your parents' love for you?
- Do you think of yourself as having grown up in a warm, loving environment?

THAT TIME OF THE MONTH

Getting your period may be one of the more memorable times in your life. Beginning menstruation is an important milestone. It marks the entry into womanhood, enabling you to give birth to another life. It's the first sign that you are an adult woman and it's one of the first major signs of puberty, along with breast development and growth of pubic hair.

How your parents reacted when you told them the news likely affected your sexual response later on. If your experience was shrouded in shame, and talked about in secret, implying it had to be hidden, it may have caused you to have negative feelings about your body. If that entry into sexuality was tainted by negative reactions by the people whom you respected, you may have internalized those negative feelings. Often it's the reason why women feel badly about their genitals, feel dirty and unattractive when menstruating, and want to avoid sexual contact.

Of course, parental reactions vary greatly. Upon menstruation, some girls' mothers took them to celebrate with an ice cream sundae, whereas others had no one to tell, knowing their mother wouldn't have been emotionally or physically available. Some women report they had no idea why they were bleeding and thought maybe they were deathly ill. If it's explained clearly, acknowledged as a milestone, it helps you to develop good feelings about your body. There doesn't have to be a twenty-one-gun salute, but without an understanding of what it is and how to manage your period, you really may think your period is a "curse." For many women it contributes to a negative genital self-image and negative body image entirely.

Timing Is Everything

Do you remember how old you were when you first got your period? Most women do. The age a girl begins menstruating affects her sexuality later on. It can be traumatizing to get your period too early or too late. If you are the first on your block to get your period and develop breasts, you may have suffered from:

Negative attention. Being first isn't always best. Singled out as the girl who got her period can make you self-conscious. It can have your body associated with humiliation. Early taunts about your body can be devastating and have long-lasting consequences.

If you got your period later than your friends, you may have felt that you were ill. Getting your period much later than your friends may have been alarming—making you feel there was something wrong with you, especially if your mom, or someone at home, didn't reassure you that it was normal. Maybe you suffered in silence. But if you got your period later than your peers, and talked to your mother about it, and perhaps learned that she didn't begin menstruating until she was fifteen or sixteen, it probably provided immediate relief. But without that outlet, you might have felt abnormal and fearful you would never develop.

In the Dark:
Diane's Story

When Diane, who is now in her seventies, got her period, she was completely in the dark as to what was happening to her body. Sex and female anatomy were taboo subjects in her home. When she began to menstruate she thought she was dying. She didn't feel comfortable asking her mother because it was clear she wasn't available for body-related questions. So Diane didn't know what was going on until much later, when after getting a few periods and crying herself to sleep, she finally asked a friend.

For years that initial trauma stuck with her, and she always associated her period with something shameful. Diane was well into adulthood before she could openly accept and discuss anything related to her period.

A Cause for Celebration:
Robin's Story

On the other hand, when Robin, now in her forties, got her period, her mother was thrilled. She called her friends to spread the good news, bought a cake, took her out for a special dinner, and even cried with joy and pride. At first Robin was horrified with her mother's behavior and felt she was a bit extreme. Robin was sure that her mother was overreacting. But growing up she felt proud of her child-bearing ability, and felt good about her body and her sexuality because the environment she grew up in embraced that milestone.

Berman Footnote

For a lot of women who have extreme bloating during their period, weight gain, pain, heavy bleeding, or even PMS (premenstrual syndrome), they associate their body with unpleasantness. Also, menstrual cycles vary—what's normal for one woman is abnormal for another. Erratic periods, getting your period late, or skipping a month here or there doesn't mean you won't be able to give birth. Before jumping to conclusions, check with your doctor.

QUESTIONS

- How old were you when you began menstruating?
- How did you feel the first time you menstruated?
- Did many of your friends begin menstruating before you did, or were you one of the first in your crowd?
- Who was the first person you told?
- What was her or his reaction?
- If the first person wasn't a parent, then how did your parents react when you told them?
- Were you prepared for how to handle it?

- **Did your culture or religion have an impact on your feelings about menstruation?**

SEXUAL MESSAGES

Women often tell Laura that growing up they had the impression that their parents rarely if ever had sex. They say: "I know they had sex twice to have my brother and me, but there was no sexual energy or real affection. It was clearly an asexual environment." Other women may say: "Of course my parents didn't have sex in front of us, but they were very warm toward one another, and their door would be locked on Sunday morning, and we knew what they were doing. They would flirt with each other and there was a lot of sexual energy between them."

Parents don't realize how great an influence this has on their children. They believe if they hide their sexuality from their children they are protecting them, but in reality it's the opposite. A lot of women worry that if they put a lock on their door their kids will know what's going on. But it's healthy for kids to know that their parents have a sex life, because it's positively modeling for them that a sexual relationship is part of a good marriage or partnership.

Messages get passed down to children. Often women come of age with negative messages about sex because their mother didn't like sex. Your mother's attitude toward sexuality shapes who you are as a woman, and sometimes in a very unconscious way. If your mother felt badly about her body, chances are you are pretty hard on your body, too. If your mother complained that all men want is sex, or confided in you that she didn't want sex but your father pressured her, or even communicated that sex was a way to get a piece of jewelry, that's what you may have grown up believing.

- What was the general attitude toward sex in your home, spoken or unspoken?
- Did you grow up believing that your mother didn't like having sex?
- Did your mother confide in you about her sex life, or lack of one?
- Did you grow up thinking your parents had an active sex life?
- Did your parents have their private time?

INAPPROPRIATE BEHAVIOR

Even the most well-meaning parents can sometimes cross the line, but when parents fail to maintain appropriate boundaries or roles, it has a profound impact on their children. To begin with, parents should not put their child into the role of caretaker or confidant. When parents share their sexual woes with their child it's unhealthy not only for the parent, but for the child as well. Sometimes mothers and fathers will confide in their children because they are too uncomfortable telling their friends and they don't want to get professional help. But when children are exposed to their parents' sexual conflicts, they feel confused, overwhelmed, and sometimes even stimulated. They don't yet have an understanding or comprehension of adult sexuality, and hearing tales by either parent can prove to be frightening.

What else can overstep parent/child boundaries? Habitually bringing your child into bed with you. But an exhausted mother or father can't always think clearly. A rash of sleepless nights can cloud anyone's judgment. The typical scenario is the baby wakes up crying for mommy and daddy, and wanting to comfort their child, the parents bring the baby into their bed. Before long, a habit is formed. This habit becomes ingrained and takes so much energy to break. At two in the morning everyone is too tired to deal with a change, hoping that the child will outgrow it and thinking it's a harmless gesture.

However, if parents allow their child to sleep in their bed on a regular basis, especially while they are having sex, it can create problems.

At some point the child will become titillated or uneasy seeing her mother and father naked or scantily clothed or even making love. Parents may think their child is unaware of what's going on, but that might not be the case. The bedroom should be the domain of the parents and not the family. That's an important model for the child to grow up with.

In some cultures families don't have the luxury of having separate bedrooms for their children, but in the United States, it's the norm. For some couples, keeping the child in bed is a way to avoid sex altogether.

QUESTIONS

- **Did you sleep in your parents' bed when you were little?**
- **If so, until what age?**
- **Did you get the impression that your parents were having sex?**
- **Did you feel that either your mother or your father used you as an excuse to avoid sex?**

FATHERLY LOVE

Were you daddy's little girl? If so, you probably feel comfortable around the opposite sex. There is no doubt that the relationship a daughter has with her father shapes how she forms other male relationships throughout her life. A girl's experience with her mother is one where she models herself after her and bonds with her. But in her relationship with her father there is not that identification; instead, her father becomes her first experience of how the rest of the world, especially men, see her.

See where you fit into these different father-daughter relationships, and how they leave their mark:

The apple of his eye. This father is affectionate, positive, complimentary, and loving. This is how the daughter then experiences herself in the outside world. As she gets older, the way her father feels about her represents the way all men will feel about her. When a man notices special features that her father recognized and cherished, whether it be her eyes, hair, intelligence, or sense of humor, she will feel attracted to him. That's a big part of what allows her to fall in love. The value her father places on her is the value she expects from other men in her life. Since her father treats her well with love, adoration, and respect, she has those expectations as she moves forward and builds romantic relationships with other men.

Too busy to bond. This father is unavailable, works late, or is off socializing with friends and doesn't spend time with his daughter. The daughter feels rejected and it becomes internalized. She may develop poor self-esteem and have difficulty trusting men. A totally absent father, too, can play a role in the daughter's sexuality. However, many girls without a father in the home connect with another male, perhaps an uncle, grandfather, teacher, or coach, because they crave that male connection. If you were raised without a father in the home, it doesn't mean you are guaranteed to enter into unhealthy relationships. But you may enter into intense, romantic relationships too readily.

A study by psychologist Bruce J. Ellis, at the University of Canterbury in New Zealand, found that teenage girls with absentee fathers tend to engage in early sexual activity and get pregnant more often than girls who were raised in homes with fathers. The study involved 242 girls living in the United States and 520 girls living in Christchurch, New Zealand.

Just plain mean. This relationship is defined by abuse. The father is cruel, critical, controlling, and maybe even violent. Unfortunately, those damaging qualities are what the daughter seeks in relationships later in life. If the father is an alcoholic, she is more likely to wind up with an alcoholic partner. If her father is insulting and/or physically abusive, she may wind up with a man who is abusive. When women look for father figures, it doesn't necessarily mean someone who is a lot older; it can just be someone authoritative or very controlling.

When a father is cruel or dismissive, the daughter may begin to act out sexually and become promiscuous because she is looking for male intimacy and closeness. When she starts to get male attention, even if it's in the form of sex, it feels better to her than no attention at all. She may go from one unsatisfying relationship to another simply searching for male affection.

Looking Back at Dad

In evaluating your relationship with your father, you want to think about how your father treated you as you went through puberty. Some fathers encourage and support their daughter's sexual development as she grows breasts and becomes a woman. Other fathers become anxious as their daughter matures, are uncomfortable with her sexuality, and are no longer affectionate with her. Some fathers react strongly to their daughter when she is fashionably dressed in revealing attire and tight jeans. They try to bully their daughter because her sexual development is so anxiety-provoking for them.

Repercussions of a Father's Temper: Rebecca's Story

Rebecca, thirty-two years old, wasn't able to maintain a relationship with a man until she was almost thirty years old. Her father, although he acted lovingly toward her, had an explosive temper. Because his behavior was unpredictable, she was afraid to be around him. This translated to being timid and withdrawn around men. It wasn't until she went into therapy that she connected the fear of men to the fear of being around her father. She is now engaged to be married.

Getting Attention the Hard Way:
Catherine's Story

Catherine's father gave her appearance and sexuality a lot of attention. As she entered adolescence she found the only time she got his attention was when she was dressed in tight, revealing clothing. She came to believe that the only way she was worthwhile was if she was flirtatious or wore skimpy clothes. Catherine's father was sexually inappropriate, even engaging in sex with his extramarital affair in her bedroom. Catherine started sleeping around with random partners in order to attract attention, and ended up getting into sexual relationships with people who mistreated her. This deeply affected her self-esteem because the only way she experienced herself positively in men's eyes was as a sexual object. She began to feel like damaged goods, and lost all self-respect.

It wasn't until she completely lost interest in doing anything fun that she realized it was time to get help. Catherine entered into therapy, confronted her father about how he treated her, and eventually she began to feel better about herself. She is now happily married with children.

QUESTIONS

- Were you close to your father growing up?
- Was your father critical or judgmental?
- What kind of relationship did you have with your father?
- Did your father encourage and support your sexual development?
- Was he available for questions or comments?
- Did you feel loved by him or did you fear the loss of his love?
- Was he punishing when you dressed in a way he considered provocative?

MOTHERLY LOVE

Just as powerful as the relationship between father and daughter is the connection between mother and daughter. As we said, a girl's mother is her model. If the mother is self-assured and empowered, the daughter often feels the same way. If the mother is meek and fearful, the child may develop similarly. A mother's comfort with her own body also is transmitted to her daughter, helping her to develop positive sexual feelings about herself.

See where you fit into these mother-daughter relationships, and how it leaves its mark:

Unconditional love. The mother's love toward her daughter is absolute, no matter what. She is supportive, protective, loving, nonjudgmental—all of which help build self-esteem and the roots of a healthy sex life.

Constantly critical. On the other hand, if the mother is uncaring and fault-finding, the daughter internalizes these messages, her self-esteem is shattered, and she often becomes insecure and pulls back emotionally, not to mention sexually.

Bossy and dominant. When a mother is domineering and/or controlling, the daughter often develops a poor self-image and can become withdrawn and shy, allowing herself to be dominated. When the daughter grows up, however, she may start acting out and rebelling, and ultimately feel guilty about her negative behavior. If this happens, it does not mean the daughter begins to feel empowered; rather, she is trying to break away from the dominance. If a child never gets a chance to feel powerful, in control, efficacious, smart, attractive, and capable, she will have a hard time developing autonomy and the necessary qualities to become sexually empowered.

The mother may also want to squelch her daughter's sexuality. It can be because she fears for her daughter's safety and virtue, or because she longs for or resents her daughter's developing sexual energy and the attention she receives. Then the mother becomes competitive and does not encourage her daughter's healthy sexual development.

My Mother Is My Competition: Nancy's Story

Nancy, a woman in her early fifties, came to see Laura because she was struggling with body image and self-esteem issues and had a hard time asserting herself sexually. Growing up, her mother was sexually competitive with her. Whenever Nancy would have male friends over, her mother would come into the room in skimpy little outfits and flirt with the boys. Sometimes her mother, who was relatively young and attractive, would even stroke her boyfriends on their back and shoulders. Nancy came of age feeling unsafe to explore her own sexuality and sexual attractiveness, feeling it meant competing with her mother. She felt she didn't have a safe place within her family structure. Not only was it damaging because of issues of trust and boundaries, it affected her confidence and personality.

She wound up doing the reverse when she reached adulthood. If anyone flirted with her she turned away. She was very uncomfortable getting any sexual attention. She was the opposite of her mother with her own daughters, but by doing that she wasn't a great role model.

Nancy was able to look back and trace where, when, and how her problems began, and tried hard to break old habits. She made a special effort not to withdraw when her daughters brought male friends and lovers home. It wasn't an easy habit to break, but she did it.

QUESTIONS

- Was your mother critical or complimentary and supportive?
- What messages did she give you about how a woman should behave sexually?
- Was your mother domineering or controlling?
- Do you think your mother was envious of your youth?
- Was your mother competitive with you for male attention?

SIBLING RELATIONSHIPS

We have all heard the stories. Big sister is happy as a lark until mommy and daddy bring home that little unwanted surprise package—baby brother. It's from that day on that sibling rivalry takes place. So it's no wonder that how your parents treated you in regard to your siblings, and how you interacted with your siblings, will affect your self-esteem and confidence. If your siblings received more attention, were told they were smarter or more attractive, then it can impair how you feel about yourself.

If you have a sister and she is favored over you, your relationship can take on a competitive tone. At different stages of your lives you may compete for the affection of your parents, friends, relatives, and even potential mates. This competition doesn't end when sisters grow up and leave the house; it can be carried on throughout their whole lives.

If any of your siblings got into any trouble because of sex, for example, they contracted a sexually transmitted disease, got pregnant, were raped or sexually molested, it would create a lot of anxiety and inhibitions in regards to sex, or even cause embarrassment or shame. Furthermore, if you witnessed your siblings getting into trouble for natural sexual exploration, such as masturbating or sex play, that, too, can have an impact on your sexual comfort.

Gender Bias

It may not be conscious, but some families are sexist and treat their boys and girls unequally. If a brother is favored over his sister, it may be hard for her to develop positive feelings about femininity and being a woman. As a result, she can grow up thinking she is inferior, doubting herself in relationships, in particular intimate relationships. In some countries, such as China, girls suffer great disadvantages. There have been cases where parents only want a son and if the mother gives birth to a daughter, the baby is discarded.

Even in homes where there is no male favoritism, parents tend to be more protective of their daughter, giving her restrictions they don't give their son. They may discourage or prohibit their daughter from dating until she is older, or enforce a curfew while the brother can come home at any hour. All this can hinder the girl's independence. In some families it's the daughters, not the sons, who are responsible for chores or household duties such as babysitting younger siblings, cooking, and cleaning. Parents may have different expectations, presuming the son will have more ambition, be better in math and science, and in sports. The girl, then, is saddled with low expectations and it becomes a self-fulfilling prophecy.

However, despite how the parents react to the different sexes, a brother can also be a positive male role model in a sister's life, especially if she was raised with an inattentive or absentee father. If you were close to your brother and he made you feel attractive and capable, and he was protective in a healthy way, you will likely be more trusting in future relationships with men.

When there is sexual abuse in the family, there are a lot of mixed emotions as well as guilt. When a sibling is sexually abused there is the feeling of why my brother or sister, and not me? On the one hand you are grateful that you were not the victim, on the other hand you feel guilty because you were not the one abused. Both scenarios create sexual guilt.

Favoring Her Brothers:
Jessica's Story

Jessica, age thirty-one, came from a traditional Italian family and was the only daughter of five siblings. She had two older and two younger brothers, but it was Jessica who was expected to fold laundry, do dishes, and help with the cooking. Her brothers, on the other hand, weren't expected to contribute to any of the household chores.

As if that wasn't hard enough on her, Jessica's parents enforced different social rules for her and her brothers. She wasn't allowed to date until she was eighteen, but her brothers never had an age restriction. When she did go out she had an early curfew, but her brothers could stumble into the house anytime during the night. When it came to sex, she was given very different messages from her brothers. They got pats on the back when they bragged about their latest sexual conquests; Jessica was expected to remain a virgin until she walked down the aisle with a ring on her finger. Her family drummed it into her that nice girls don't have sex before their wedding night. The message was loud and clear.

When Jessica finally did sleep with her boyfriend her senior year in college, she felt tremendous guilt. Presently she is still single, and continues to feel anxious and guilty when she engages in sex and has not been able to reach orgasm, alone or with a partner— although she is working on it.

QUESTIONS

- How would you describe your relationship with your siblings? Good, fair, or bad?
- Were they a positive influence on your self-esteem or were they a negative one?
- How did your parents handle disputes?
- Did your parents give your brother or sister preferential treatment?
- Did any of your siblings have sexually transmitted diseases, unplanned pregnancies, or other sexual troubles?

THE FIRST TIME

Not every woman thinks of intercourse when asked about her first sexual experience. Some women consider their first sexual encounter to be making out or kissing or becoming sexually aroused. But whatever you consider your first experience, if your parents became aware that you were engaging in sexual activities and were punitive or disapproving as a result, the stage might have been set for future sexual anxiety and guilt. If it was uninterrupted, natural and enjoyable, it most likely had positive implications, leaving you with a good feeling about sex.

If the first time you had sexual intercourse it was painful, awkward, or unfulfilling, you may associate intercourse with discomfort and anxiety. As a result, a vicious cycle can occur: Each time you are about to make love you anticipate the pain and become tense, which creates more pain and stress. If your first sexual experience was associated with something traumatic, you will likely carry guilt and anxiety around for a long time.

Sex and Guilt:
Marcy's Story

Marcy came from a family with very traditional values and her parents made it clear that a "good girl" doesn't have sex until she is married. She had been dating someone for a while and finally decided to have sex. But just as they were engaging in sex for the first time, the phone rang. The caller informed Marcy that her father had just died. To this day, she can't get over the guilt and feeling that, on some level, her having sex was connected to her father's death. She is now in her thirties and has been carrying that guilt around, unable to enjoy sex.

Needless to say, if you have sex for the first time and are later rejected, it can have a big impact on your sexual future. When a girl gives of herself fully only to be cast aside afterward, a myriad of problems can follow. Typically, she feels used, misled, and discarded, causing her to feel unsafe. She no longer trusts her judgment. Worse yet, if word gets out in school that she had sex and her classmates taunt her, she will feel even more vulnerable, ostracized, and likely to develop guilt, shame, and anxiety about sex.

Being branded the "school slut" or "easy" is devastating for high school girls. In *Fast Girls*, author Emily White talks about how quickly rumors spread, how one day girls were part of the crowd and the next day a target.

When a girl offers her virginity to a boy in order to keep him and he drops her after they have sex, a few things can happen. She can feel duped and ashamed and become less trusting in future relationships. Or she may feel that since she has already lost her virginity she may as well sleep around, having meaningless sex with lots of partners. Ultimately, the more control and success you had with that first experience, the better off your sex life will be.

If a girl's first sexual experience was a positive one in a good relationship, it's just another stage in her sexual development. But if she has sex for the wrong reasons, such as peer pressure, or to hold on to her boyfriend, or just because she wanted to get it over with, and it was a bad experience, it will negatively impact future relationships and how she feels about sex in general.

QUESTIONS

- What was your first sexual experience?
- Was it pleasurable or stressful?
- What inspired you to have sex the first time?
- Was it something you planned or was it spontaneous?
- How did your partner treat you afterward? What was the aftereffect?
- Was the first time associated with anything traumatic?

SEXUAL ORIENTATION

Many women have had some sort of homosexual fantasy, and it's not uncommon to have a crush on another person of the same sex sometime in your life. Whether it's because you admire a particular woman, aspire to be like her, or are intrigued by her, there are many shades of gray. But that doesn't mean you are a lesbian. It's a natural part of development. If growing up you had a little sex play with a girlfriend, such as kissing or touching, this, too, is natural. But many women who were caught in the act by their caregivers were scolded, punished, or humiliated. This overreaction can blow the incident way out of proportion and create tremendous guilt and apprehension regarding sex.

Similarly, if a woman grows up preferring females, and is forced or pressured to be heterosexual by her parents or peers when her heart isn't in it, all kinds of conflicts are created with regard to her sexual satisfaction. She might feel anxious about her sexual preferences, have difficulty responding sexually, find it hard to commit to a sexual relationship with another woman, and feel the need to hide her sexual preferences.

QUESTIONS

- **Did you ever engage in sex play with other girls?**
- **Were you ever discovered and what was the reaction you received?**
- **If you were attracted to women growing up, did your parents discourage you from preferring women?**

A TRAUMA HISTORY

Without a doubt, children who have been physically, emotionally, or sexually abused pay a very hefty price. From this trauma, they may develop any number of the following:

Depression

Sleep disturbances

Eating disorders

Difficulty trusting people

Poor self-esteem

Chronic anxiety

Substance abuse

Self-destructive behavior

Promiscuous behavior, moving from partner to partner
  indiscriminately

Poor decision-making skills regarding their sexuality, putting
  themselves at risk for STDs and HIV/AIDS

Difficulty with sexual intimacy

Poor academic record in school

Trouble bonding with peers and friends

Sexual abuse victims may also block out the incidents or suffer from flashbacks or nightmares. Often they find the shame overwhelming, and no matter how much they know that they were not responsible, there is always an element of self-blame. If the perpetrator is a family member, the child may be fearful to tell, assuming that nobody will believe her or him. It's not uncommon for a sexual abuse survivor to suffer from post-traumatic stress syndrome.

A girl who was sexually molested by a non–family member may have a better chance of overcoming the trauma if she has the support of a loving family. If the molestation took place out of the house, she will feel protected at home. But if the abuse was by a father, stepfather, brother, or uncle, she will not feel she has a "safe place" and may be at risk for even more long-term problems.

As we discussed in our book *For Women Only*, reclaiming sexuality for a woman who has suffered sexual abuse takes an enormous amount of time and work. With the help of a good therapist and supportive partner, it's possible to reach a point of resolution, accepting your past and moving on.

- Were you ever forced to have sex against your will?
- If so, was the perpetrator a relative?
- Did you tell anyone about the abuse?
- If so, what was their reaction? Did he or she believe you?
- If the perpetrator was a stranger, did you find comfort at home with your family?
- Did or do you have nightmares or flashbacks about the abuse?

Healing

Overcoming the effects of childhood abuse, undoing the emotional damage, and going on with a productive secure life isn't easy. Treatment for sexual abuse involves different stages of healing and recovery, and is not a short process. Trust lost in childhood is not easy to regain. But history can't be changed, and you can only move forward. Here are steps in healing:

Acknowledge the abuse. The wish to repress and deny painful memories is very strong, but accepting your past is essential to healing. In *The Courage to Heal*, Ellen Bass and Laura Davis point out that trust is learned in childhood, but when a child is abused, that trust is broken. When sexual abuse occurs, trust and intimacy are filled with anxiety, and relationships are difficult to develop and maintain.

Resolve the memories and painful feelings. The memories sometimes come back in flashbacks and nightmares. They are often painful and terrifying to recount, but in a warm and supportive treatment setting, these memories and associated feelings can be expressed and detoxified of their debilitating effects. Feelings of anger, betrayal, guilt, humiliation, anxiety, and shame often occur and need to be talked about. There is anger at the perpetrator, and sometimes with yourself for allowing it to happen. If the abuse has been by a parent or if caretakers did not protect you enough, the feelings of betrayal and anger are often directed at parents and caretakers as well.

Eventually, by working through these destructive emotions in a trusting, caring relationship, the feelings will dissipate and be replaced by trust and a desire for intimacy. Support groups with other survivors of sexual abuse can also be very helpful.

Moving on. Allow yourself to enter into a healthy relationship. This means redefining your sexuality on your terms, learning how to trust again, and gaining the courage to find intimacy in a relationship, sexual and otherwise.

BOTTOM LINE

Getting to the root of your hang-ups, uneasiness, fears, or phobias about sex can free you to have a sexually satisfied life. Oftentimes we feel or behave a certain way without knowing why, but exploring and confronting your past can only help. And looking into your history doesn't mean dredging up bad memories, either. You are bound to have wonderful recollections, fond feelings, and loving moments that will make you feel good, too.

Accepting and Overcoming Physical Obstacles

Just as you need to address past life experiences, you need to look into medical problems that can affect your sex life. We would be remiss if we ignored your physical health. In fact, we find that sexually satisfied women do everything in their power to preempt medical problems. No, they are not immune to coming down with a disease or illness, but they tackle whatever medical obstacle they en-

FINDINGS FROM THE WOMEN'S SEXUAL SATISFACTION SURVEY

- Sexual satisfaction was related to the absence of urinary symptoms.
- Urinary leakage as a result of physical activity was related to reports of vaginal dryness.
- A greater number of urinary problems were related to dryness, low genital sensation, genital pain, and avoidance of sex.
- Menopausal women not on hormone replacement therapy have lower sexual satisfaction.
- 26 percent of women with some sort of sexual dysfunction sought help for their problem and most of them were able to resolve the problem.

counter. Therefore, this chapter is about facing whatever disability or ailment challenges you, and taking preventative measures to avoid sexual stumbling blocks because of an illness. And it's about managing your sexual health with success.

Emily's Story

It had been ten years since Emily, age fifty-two, had breast cancer. Although she was in remission and cancer free, she still suffered from low libido. Her sexual dysfunction problems started when she began her chemotherapy, but her symptoms remained long after her treatment ended. Her major complaints were, and continued to be, vaginal dryness, mood swings, depression, loss of energy, and not being able to have sex due to pain from the dryness and tightness. Emily couldn't take hormones because of the kind of breast cancer she'd had, and she wanted very badly to resume an active sex life. She came to Jennifer to find a way to get her sex life back on track.

As we age, our bodies undergo physical changes, and many of those changes can have a direct impact on our sex lives. Whether it's a natural part of aging, like menopause, or a life-threatening disease like cancer, the physiology and mechanism of sexual response can be affected. Experts agree that many health problems can prevent a woman from becoming sexually satisfied. Neurological, vascular, endocrine, and muscular illnesses or conditions can make it tough to enjoy sex, engage in sexual intercourse, or have an orgasm, not to mention cause a diminished sex drive and loss of sensation and/or lubrication. But attending to vaginal dryness, discomfort in the genital area, or any of these sex-related issues can help to improve sexual satisfaction.

Arousal requires a working vascular, muscular, and nervous system. To become aroused you need adequate blood flow, normal tissue, and a normal neurological structure. The pelvic floor muscles require strength and tone, and the clitoris, which is vascular, requires proper blood flow. The nervous system, which causes the chain of events that lead to arousal, needs to be intact in order for the blood vessels to dilate and the muscles to relax.

Many diseases and conditions produce psychological complications. Anyone suffering from a chronic and/or life-threatening illness is at risk for anxiety or depression, which are known predictors for sexual difficulties. Self-esteem, too, can be lowered, especially if there is persistent pain, which can make it hard to enjoy sex. Medications can also have an impact on the sex drive.

SEX EVERY DAY KEEPS THE DOCTOR AWAY

Just as health problems can impair your sexual functioning, it turns out that having regular sex is good for your overall health. There have been studies showing an association between an active sex life and longevity. (Of course, if you are unhealthy, not exercising, not eating well, or depressed, forcing yourself to have sex isn't the answer.) Here is what a regular dose of sex can do:

Relieve stress. Following a tough day at work or at home with the kids, having sex can calm the nerves. An active sex life is good for the heart—it gives a good aerobic workout, almost like running on the treadmill or jogging for twenty minutes. During orgasm the heart rate doubles, increasing blood flow and raising the metabolic rate.

Boost the immune system. Hormones and neurotransmitters released from the brain during sexual relations and sexual excitement help to fight against viruses, the flu, and infections. Psychologists at Wilkes University in Pennsylvania found that students who engaged in sexual activity once or twice a week had higher levels of the antibody immunoglobulin A (IgA), which boosts immune systems and fights colds and flu, than students who had sexual activity less than once a week. However, those who engaged in sex more than twice a week had lower levels of IgA. A different study conducted in Wales followed 918 men for ten years. They found that the mortality rate was 50 percent lower in the group that had frequent orgasms. All of the deaths were from heart disease.

May fight disease. There have also been claims that dehydroepiandrosterone (DHEA), a steroid hormone made from cholesterol by the adrenal glands, is released naturally at orgasm and inhibits the growth of tumors, helps bone density, and boosts the sex drive. DHEA supplements have been used to treat diabetes, heart disease, Alzheimer's, and much more. (It must be noted, however, that many doctors warn against taking the supplement, believing it can cause serious side effects.)

Can ease pain. Oxytocin, a hormone secreted by the pituitary gland in the brain, not only stimulates contractions of the uterus but also increases testosterone production and sexual sensitivity, making orgasm more powerful. Dr. Beverly Whipple, author of *The G-Spot*, found that oxytocin also has the ability to control pain. By applying pressure on the G-spot, pain can be eased, especially during vaginal stimulation and orgasm when the feel-good hormones endorphins and corticosteroids are released.

THE HORMONE CONNECTION

Hormones have a preventative role in maintaining cellular, tissue, vaginal, and skin health. The ideal time to monitor and replace missing hormones is in our late thirties and early forties, when we are perimenopausal and starting to show signs of decreasing hormones, like irritability from sleep deprivation. Suzanne Somers, in her book *The Sexy Years*, suggests starting hormones early and not waiting until the damage has been done. Somers writes that women lose 90 percent of their hormones over a two-year period once they begin menopause, and when one hormone in the system is off, the entire system is out of whack. She also believes that women who are taking synthetic hormones are not replacing the lost hormones, and recommends taking natural bioidentical hormones that replicate the hormones we make in our body. There is no "one pill fits all." Through routine blood testing we can determine which hormones we are losing and replace them gradually. For example, Somers says, a popular synthetic hormone for estrogen is Premarin, but the bioidentical one is estradiol, estrone, or estriol, which are created in a lab from plant extracts, such as soybeans.

Testosterone

Testosterone, the hormone that affects sexual desire, is considered to be the male or masculine hormone because it's associated with facial hair and a deep voice. However, women have small amounts of testosterone that are produced in the ovaries and adrenal glands, and, like estrogen, it declines gradually throughout their lives. Even women with regular menstrual periods have levels of testosterone.

We believe that testosterone is essential to a woman's sexual functioning and nothing can compensate for its absence, including intense sexual stimulation. Testosterone is essential for energy, libido, mood, and well-being.

While testosterone is not FDA approved for women yet, Procter and Gamble is presently conducting phase-three studies of a new testosterone patch. Initial testing in postmenopausal and posthysterectomized women showed promising results in increasing libido and sexual response. Testosterone is also available as an off-label prescription by your physician, who can compound doses to meet your needs. But taking testosterone or any hormone should not be done lightly. Potential side effects of testosterone include weight gain, increased cholesterol levels, liver damage (depending on the delivery), oily skin, hair growth, deepening of the voice, and enlargement of the clitoris.

MANAGED CARE

What ails you is likely to put a damper on your sex life. Unfortunately none of us have the power to ward off many of the diseases that may come our way. Making matters worse, it's not easy to have a satisfying sex life if you are riddled with pain, suffering from a chronic illness, or battling cancer or heart disease.

The following are some illnesses and conditions that interfere with sexual sensation and response—and suggestions for how to manage and enjoy an active sex life.

> **More than 64 million Americans have one or more forms of cardiovascular disease.**

Coronary Artery Disease

What it is: Coronary disease, or atherosclerosis, is a narrowing of the arteries that go to the heart muscle caused by the buildup of plaque, largely cholesterol, in these blood vessels.

When the arteries narrow there can be diminished blood flow to the heart, which can result in chest pain or angina, as the exercising heart muscle does not receive an adequate amount of blood. When a small cholesterol plaque in a coronary artery ruptures, there is a resulting deposition of blood clot on the plaque that can block the coronary artery, causing death of a portion of the heart muscle (myocardial infarction, or heart attack).

How it affects sexual response: The process of atherosclerosis—deposition of cholesterol plaques in blood vessels that leads to blockage of vessels to the heart—can also lead to blocking of vessels to the genital area.

The buildup of plaque that narrows the arteries and can cut off blood flow to the heart or brain also reduces the blood flow to the arteries that lead to the pelvis and genitalia. This causes diminished arousal in women. Blood vessels supplying the vagina need the blood flow for adequate lubrication. Ultimately, this situation can lead to vaginal dryness. The decrease in blood flow can also interfere with sexual sensation and arousal by affecting the release of nitric oxide, and can cause atrophy and degradation of the nerve fibers and cells lining the vaginal canal and inner labia. It is also not unusual for women or men who have had a heart attack, or who suffer from heart disease, to withdraw from sexual activity for fear of triggering an episode of angina. Some high-risk cardiac patients may be advised to temporarily refrain from having sex.

What to do: During recovery the doctor may advise the heart patient to abstain from intercourse, or wait until he or she has the necessary strength for sexual activity, but there are options. Other forms of intimate physical contact can be encouraged, such as holding hands, hugging, kissing, massage, use of a vibrator, mutual masturbation, and intimate verbal communication. Less active sexual positions such as semireclining, on-the-bottom, and seated positions may help reduce cardiovascular and respiratory effort. However, if the patient isn't used to varying sexual positions, this may not be the best time to try them, as heightened stimulation can increase the cardiovascular demand.

It must be noted that having coronary heart disease doesn't preclude you from having sex. As long as you are able to walk up three flights of stairs without having chest pain or becoming short of breath, you should be able to have sex. But check with your doctor.

Epilepsy

What it is: This is a neurological condition where patients experience seizures. A seizure is caused by electrical disturbances in the brain that result in a variety of symptoms depending on where the electrical disturbance occurs. It can range from a simple movement involving one extremity to a brief staring spell. If it occurs in the motor area, there may be arm movement. If it's in the sensory area, there may be visual disturbances. If it takes over the whole brain, there can be a convulsion.

How it affects sexual response: According to the Epilepsy Foundation, studies indicate that reduced sexual desire and/or sexual arousal may affect a quarter to a third of people with epilepsy. Since seizures are unpredictable, some women may be fearful that they can have an episode during sex or that sexual intercourse may bring one on. This fear can be especially overwhelming if there is a history of a seizure developing during sex. Some antiseizure medications, such as primidone and phenobarbital, may reduce sexual desire and diminish libido. The medications can cause a drop in hormones.

What to do: People with epilepsy should be able to have a normal sex life. If the antiseizure medication is causing a low sex drive, then an alternative drug should be prescribed. The worry that a seizure may occur and the concern about losing control can interfere with having a fulfilling love life. Therefore, as with any condition, discussing concerns with a partner may help ease your anxiety.

Spinal Cord Injuries

What it is: Whether it's the result of an auto accident, a fall, a sports injury, or a gunshot wound, every year thousands of Americans suffer from spinal cord injuries. Permanent loss of function occurs when the spinal cord, which runs the length of the spine, suffers from a compression injury, a break, or a shattering of the bone pressing on the spinal cord. A loss of sensation and movement in the legs and part or all of the trunk is called paraplegia, and usually involves a spinal cord injury to the mid- and lower back. A loss of sensation and movement in the arms, legs, and the trunk is quadriplegia, and usually occurs from an injury to the neck.

> Spinal cord injury affects an estimated 250,000 to 450,000 people in the United States, 18 percent of whom are women.

How it affects sexual response: A patient's mobility has a lot to do with the extent of sexual functioning. Because of the paralysis, there may be difficulty achieving certain positions, movements, and endurance. There also may be a loss of sensation. Women may suffer from arousal problems because the nerve stimulation involved in increasing genital blood flow and engorgement is injured. Women may also lose the ability to relax the vaginal muscles, and have difficulty with vaginal dryness because the stimulus that makes lubrication comes from the portion of the spinal cord that has been injured.

But Gary Karp, author of *Life on Wheels: For the Active Wheelchair*

User, says it's a myth that if a woman isn't able to compress her partner's penis in her vagina it will impair her partner's satisfaction. In fact, he says, if she isn't squeezing there is a little less friction, which means sex can last longer.

Women with adequate pelvic-floor strength and tone who can control their pelvic-floor muscles enjoy enhanced sexual arousal and pleasure for themselves, but not necessarily for their partner.

What to do: People with spinal cord injuries do not have to give up a fulfilling sex life, they just have to redefine it and change their priorities. What feels good and is attainable rises to the top of the list. If someone doesn't feel sensation during intercourse, they can still enjoy sexual contact because it's still a very intimate act, regardless if there is an orgasmic response. They need to explore their body, experiment, see what feels good and know what responses are feasible. Karp says that many people report the more delicate, subtle, sensual things become a lot more appealing, such as massage, or being licked in the erogenous zones, or deep relaxation.

For people with a spinal cord injury, grieving the loss and expressing their feelings is very important. But achieving sexual satisfaction will be difficult if they dwell on how things used to be. While the emotional impact is great, the key is being with a trusting partner. It may take some time, but in working together a fulfilling sex life can be obtained.

Migraine Headaches

> 3 out of 4 migraine sufferers are women.
> 18 percent of women experience migraine headaches.

What it is: Migraine headaches are characterized by severe, intense, throbbing and debilitating head pain. The headache can attack just one side of the head and be accompanied by nausea, vomiting, dizziness, and sensitivity to light and noise. Migraines can begin with or without an aura, which is the occurrence of flashing lights, zigzag lines, or temporary loss of vision, as well as other neurological symptoms. An aura usually presents ten to forty-five minutes before onset of the headache, and occurs in only about 15 percent of patients.

Women are more likely to suffer from a migraine than men, and experts believe it's due to the fluctuation of hormone levels. The estrogen hormone influences the brain receptors of migraine-prone people, making them more vulnerable. Migraines can also be triggered upon menstruation. Some women prone to migraines are likely to develop them the first two days before their period begins, the day of onset, or the day after. Some women develop a migraine exclusively during their period and at no other time of the month. While most migraines are severe, at times a migraine can present as a mild headache, or even just an aura without any headache.

How it affects sexual response: Headaches in general may have a relationship to orgasm or sexual excitement, according to migraine specialist Joel Saper at the Michigan Head Pain and Neurological Institute in Ann Arbor, Michigan. A headache may occur just prior to, at the time of, or just after orgasm, he says. Orgasm itself can trigger a headache, which has even been noted during masturbation. This is possibly related to the neurotransmitter rush, such as release of dopamine, serotonin, or norepinephrine.

Although it is possible that worrying about making love can bring on a headache, for some people, just exerting themselves during sex can cause a headache, or even make an existing one worse. An exertion headache can continue during sexual activity, cease when sexual activity stops, or develop into a complete migraine. Certain postures during sex can also bring on a migraine. The physical straining of the neck, arching of the back, or straining of the jaw can cause pounding, debilitating head pain. (All cases of severe headache with exertion or otherwise should be examined by a physician, to rule out anything serious.) Headache can be associated with a loss of incentive, since someone suffering from a pounding headache will hardly be in the mood for sexual excitement.

What to do: Some headache-prone people take nonsteroid or over-the-counter drugs, like Motrin or Aleve, before they have sex to prevent a headache from coming on. Doctors may prescribe prescription drugs as a precautionary measure, such as Midrin, sumatriptan (Imitrex), rizatriptan (Maxalt), zolmitriptan (Zomig), and almotriptan (Axert). Some headache sufferers may prefer to take the medication only on the weekends, which are prime sexual times. If the headache seems to be related to posture, then sexual positions need to be modified—for example, engaging in positions that cause less straining of the neck or back. Pacing oneself can also be helpful, allowing for less physical stress. Perhaps a slower buildup and longer foreplay. When someone feels a headache coming on, they should stop and take a break.

Sleep Disorders

What it is: According to the National Sleep Foundation about 70 million people in the United States have difficulty sleeping. The American Academy of Sleep Medicine found that women are twice as likely as men to have a tough time falling and staying asleep. Perhaps it's because there is a higher incidence of anxiety and depression in women, which is associated with insomnia, or a drop in hormone levels. Many experts believe that sleeplessness, very common in our perimenopausal and menopausal patients, is related to insufficient estrogen. However, stress, anxiety, and depression can all affect sleep patterns as well.

Reasons why people have trouble falling asleep vary. Those with daytime worries typically bring them to bed at night, making it difficult to relax and let sleep take over. Grieving over the loss of a loved one makes it hard to fall asleep, as do medical problems such as cancer, arthritis, chronic pain, and osteoporosis. Pregnancy and changes in the menstrual cycle, such as menopause and nighttime hot flashes, can also disrupt sleep.

More serious conditions, such as sleep apnea, narcolepsy, and restless leg syndrome, can be the reason. Sleep apnea is a breathing disorder in which the patient wakes up gasping for breath during the night. It's potentially life-threatening and is characterized by snoring and excessive daytime sleepiness. Narcolepsy is excessive and overwhelming daytime sleepiness, regardless of how much sleep is obtained at night. Sufferers can fall asleep anywhere, including while eating, driving, or talking. Restless leg syndrome is a very uncomfortable creepy, crawly sensation inside the leg that occurs during the day. Patients feel agitated and have difficulty remaining still. At night, many sufferers have periodic limb movement disorder in which there is a slight twitch of the muscles of the lower leg every one to two minutes. This movement disrupts sleep.

How it affects sexual response: There is data in men that normal REM (rapid eye movement) sleep is needed to maintain an erection. There is also a study indicating that women can get clitoral erections during REM sleep. Normal sleep is important to maintain genital blood flow. Sleep disturbances affect mood, energy, and memory, and if any of those things are out of whack, your desire to be sexual will be diminished.

What to do: Being sleep deprived can affect one's overall energy as well as sexual energy. To get a good night's sleep, try the following measures:

- Avoid alcohol, caffeine, and nicotine within a few hours of bedtime.
- Put bills and disagreements aside. Inflammatory discussions will keep you tossing and turning.

- Exercise, but not before bedtime. Avoid working out three hours before bedtime, as it will stimulate you.
- Create a restful environment. Make it uncluttered and use comfortable pillows and blankets. Eliminate offending noise.
- Establish a regular sleeping pattern. Try going to bed and waking up the same time each day.

Autoimmune Diseases: Rheumatoid Arthritis

2.1 million Americans suffer from rheumatoid arthritis; 70 percent of people with RA are women.

What it is: This is a systemic inflammatory autoimmune disease that occurs when the immune system attacks the healthy tissues lining the joints, called the synovium. This causes an inflammation that can damage the cartilage and bone in the fingers, hips, knees, ankles, feet, wrists, and neck. When this happens, swelling, tenderness, stiffness, redness, and discomfort can result. Patients can also develop fever, fatigue, weight loss, and nodules under the skin.

How it affects sexual response: People with arthritis can have difficulty enjoying sex mostly because of pain in the hip, not because of low sexual desire. Other than pain, there can be limited hip movement, which makes intercourse uncomfortable. Some people develop erosion of the joints and cartilage, causing obvious deformity. Treatment can include steroids, which can cause weight gain and a bloated appearance. When physical appearance is altered, low self-esteem, inhibition, and insecurity can develop. As we have discussed, if someone doesn't feel good about the way they look, they may avoid intimacy.

What to do: If there is restricted movement in the hip or joints, or certain positions during intercourse are uncomfortable or painful, then new positions should be explored. Positions involving weight-bearing and a lot of movement can be problematic. Pillows may be needed to protect sensitive joints. Sometimes taking pain medication before engaging in sexual activity can alleviate any potential discomfort.

The Arthritis Foundation offers a *Guide to Intimacy*, suggesting different positions that can be comfortable—minimizing the pain—and enjoyable during sex. (See the Appendix for where to get a copy.) A few of their lovemaking suggestions include the following:

- **Both partners lie on their sides and the man enters from behind. If a woman has hip problems, she can try putting a pillow between her knees. Good for hip problems.**
- **The women kneels with her upper body supported by furniture or pillows. Good for hip problems.**
- **The woman lies on her back with both knees flexed. This is good for women whose tendons or muscles are severely shortened.**
- **Both partners stand. The man enters from behind. The woman leans on furniture at a comfortable height for support and balance. Good for anyone who has difficulty in a kneeling position.**

Diabetes

An estimated 13 million Americans have been diagnosed with diabetes. About 5.2 million people are unaware they have the disease.

What it is: Diabetes is the result of an insufficient production of insulin, which is a hormone produced by cells in the pancreas. Insulin helps the body process sugar and carbohydrates. There are two major kinds of diabetes: Type 1 is when the pancreas fails to make enough insulin and mostly strikes people under the age of thirty. Type 2, most common after age forty, is when the pancreas may produce insulin but the body is unable to adequately respond to it. There is also a third, temporary type of diabetes called gestational diabetes, which develops during pregnancy but usually disappears after the birth of the child.

Patients with diabetes have the potential for developing kidney failure, heart disease, stroke, nerve damage, and blindness. These complications occur when the insulin blocks glucose from entering cells and causes it to build up in the bloodstream. Experts in the field believe that some people have a predisposition to diabetes, and once they reach a certain weight beyond their normal body weight, they are likely to develop Type 2. Speculation about causes for Type 1 center around a viral trigger in those who are genetically predisposed. It is a myth that eating sweets can cause the disease.

How it affects sexual response: Diabetics often have high levels of cholesterol in their blood, which can diminish blood flow to their sex organs. When this occurs there is a lack of lubrication. A study comparing 120 women with diabetes and 180 healthy women, reported in the April 2002 issue of *Diabetes Care*, found decreased sexual arousal and reduced vaginal lubrication in women with diabetes. A decreased sexual desire and pain during intercourse due to vaginal dryness may also be experienced by women with diabetes.

High levels of glucose in the vaginal mucus can make women prone to yeast infections, which can cause discomfort during sex. Although diabetes does not cause low libido in women, women with the disease tend to have more sexual function complaints than those without it. Medications can be the root of the problem, or they might be suffering from depression, which makes them disinterested in sex.

What to do: Keeping blood sugar under control can help prevent complications that lead to sexual problems. Dryness can be addressed by using lubricants or estrogen replacement. It's possible that the insulin or medication needs to be adjusted. If medication and diet are under control, sexual response should be normal.

Cancer

What it is: The American Cancer Society (ACS) describes cancer as "a group of diseases characterized by uncontrolled growth and spread of abnormal cells." The ASC estimates that 1,368,030 new cancer cases are expected to be diagnosed in 2004. (These numbers do not include basal and squamous cell skin cancers and noninvasive cancer of any site except the urinary bladder.) The most prevalent cancers in women (in order) are breast, lung and bronchus, colon and rectal, uterine and ovarian.

Other than surgical removal of the cancerous tumor, treatment often involves chemotherapy and/or radiation. Chemotherapy utilizes a group of potent, toxic chemicals designed to kill malignant cells. While it destroys the cancer, it also harms healthy cells. Other than hair loss and nausea, chemotherapy can cause hormone levels to drop dramatically and cause anemia and low white cell counts. Radiation, or X-ray therapy, involves high doses of radioactive waves that penetrate the tumor. The purpose is to stop the growth of cancer cells. Both radiation therapy and chemotherapy can cause great fatigue through their effects in part on lowering red and white cell counts.

Dealing with cancer can take a psychological, emotional, and physical toll. The fear and stress of being stricken with a life-threatening illness can diminish a patient's sexual desire. Battling a potentially deadly disease can lead to depression and anxiety, which are not conducive to an active sex life. Exhaustion from radiation, a loss of estrogen and progesterone from surgical removal of the ovaries, and toxicity from chemotherapy can all alter sexual functioning.

How it affects sexual response: Generally, the impact of cancer on sexual response depends on the type of cancer and course of treatment. Most affected are gynecological cancers treated by surgery and/or radiation and chemotherapy. In fact, any cancer that requires chemotherapy can result in sexual difficulties as the treatment typically puts women into menopause. Pelvic surgery can involve removal of the uterus, cervix, ovaries, bladder, and fallopian tubes. Vulva surgery can involve the clitoris and inner and outer lips.

We have noticed that women who had a hysterectomy (removal of the uterus, cervix, and possibly ovaries) have a decrease in vaginal sensations and libido and difficulty reaching orgasm. If the ovaries get a high dose of radiation, they stop making hormones. Without estrogen, there is vaginal dryness and loss of the blood supply and elasticity of the vagina. When radiation hits the vaginal area directly, it can cause scarring and intercourse becomes tight or painful because the vagina is dry and doesn't stretch out with sexual arousal.

Although it's uncommon, some women undergoing radiation develop painful vaginal ulcers that don't heal. When there is intense radiation, the walls and lining of the vagina can stick together, which can be prevented by regular intercourse or by using a vaginal dilator.

Long-term sexual problems often occur in women who had chemotherapy for breast cancer. If they are in their forties or younger, it puts them into menopause immediately, prematurely and permanently, giving them all the sexual problems related to menopause, such as vaginal dryness and vaginal atrophy due to the lack of estrogen.

Some women who have a mastectomy or gynecological surgery become self-conscious, and feel that they have lost their sex appeal, which can cause them to withdraw. Following a mastectomy, some women develop chronic pain or pressure in the chest and shoulders, which makes getting into certain positions difficult. For many women their breasts are a means of sexual stimulation, and this is a loss.

What to do: It is expected that there will be some difficulty with sexual response following cancer treatment. For emotional support, women with cancer should be patient and communicate their feelings to their partner. If vaginal dryness is a problem, a water-based lubricant can be used. If there is pain with intercourse, the doctor may suggest a local form of estrogen or a vaginal dilator or gynecological physical therapy.

Women with breast cancer can't take hormones, and studies are currently in progress to test for safe and effective treatments for vaginal dryness. If their cancer is estrogen positive, hormones can't be prescribed. Viagra might help, as well as the other nonhormonal arousal enhancers.

WOMEN ONLY

Menopause

What it is: It was once only whispered about, and referred to as "the change." But women no longer keep menopause a secret. Thanks to an overabundance of articles, web information, and TV talk shows, menopause, the cessation of a woman's menstrual periods, is out in the open. It may mean the end of a woman's reproductive years, but it is not an affliction, is nothing to be ashamed of, and is a natural progression of the female aging process. Although a woman can reach menopause in her thirties or forties, average age is about fifty-one. Menopause is usually gradual and begins years earlier with irregular periods and a change in the normal menstrual cycle. A woman may have a lighter or heavier bleeding of longer or shorter duration, or skip periods altogether. Symptoms include hot flashes or a drenching perspiration during the night called night sweats. There can also be heart palpitations, where the heart feels like it's beating erratically or fast, a thinning of the hair or loss of elasticity in the skin, mood swings, incontinence, and depression.

How it affects sexual response: When a woman reaches menopause there is a dramatic drop of estrogen produced in her ovaries. (It's this loss of estrogen that causes the symptoms, such as hot flashes.) When this happens, the tissues of the vagina and vulva become thin and dry. It's the production of estrogen that keeps a woman lubricated. The loss of estrogen not only causes a decrease in vaginal secretions, but can also cause irritation, inflammation, and vaginal atrophy. Many menopausal women struggle with symptoms of low testosterone as well, including low libido, low energy, and difficulty responding sexually. Testosterone does not drop off as sharply as estrogen does with menopause. Most women notice the symptoms of low testosterone while they are still in perimenopause, the years prior to menopause when hormonal fluctuations begin and menstrual irregularity sets in.

What to do: Menopause doesn't mean the end of your sex life. For years, millions of women took hormone replacement therapy (HRT) to ease the symptoms of menopause and help prevent osteoporosis and heart disease. But following the bombshell from some studies, including the Women's Health Initiative, there has been controversy about using HRT. The studies found that Prempro, a combination of estrogen and progesterone, increased the risk of heart disease, blood clots, and stroke. This left many women across America searching for an alternative treatment. Even before the WHI study, it was recommended that women with breast cancer, or with a strong family history of the disease, avoid HRT, as breast cancers can be stimulated by estrogens.

Menopause management needs to be individually tailored to meet each woman's needs. There is no blanket therapy. Since there are some advantages to hormone therapies, women should check with their doctor. Symptoms, side effects, risk factors, and family history should all be taken into consideration. Here are some other options: Raloxifene (Evista) is used to treat and prevent osteoporosis (decreased density of bone mass) in postmenopausal women. It is not an estrogen or hormone therapy; it's what is known as a selective estrogen receptor modulator (SERM). In addition to treating osteoporosis, raloxifene has been shown to reduce the chances of developing breast cancer and to prevent bone loss at the hip, spine, and rest of the body. Side effects include hot flashes, leg cramps, and increased risk of deep-vein thrombosis (blood clots). Raloxifene does not help treat vaginal atrophy or hot flashes.

As we have discussed, lubricating gels will help the dryness. Vaginal and testosterone estrogen cream can also help dryness. Estrogen creams do get absorbed into the body, although not as much as when estrogen is taken orally. Other choices include:

- **ESTRING:** a soft ring inserted into the vagina that releases a low dose of estrogen for ninety days.
- **FEMRING:** a silicone ring inserted into the vagina that releases a low dose of estrogen for three months at a time.
- **VAGIFEM:** a vaginal estrogen tablet inserted with a disposable applicator. It releases a continuous low dose of estrogen into the vaginal tissue to relieve dryness and irritation.

Myths and Facts about Menopause

Pick up any number of women's magazines and you are bound to come across tips on how to tackle the symptoms of menopause. But even with the wealth of information available, there are still some misconceptions. Here are three common myths and facts:

MYTH: Menopause doesn't occur until after age fifty.
FACT: Many women go into menopause in their thirties and forties, either naturally or induced as a result of a hysterectomy or removal of the ovaries.

MYTH: Every woman experiences hot flashes.
FACT: While hot flashes are certainly common, women can have numerous symptoms to hardly any.

MYTH: When you are starting to skip periods and in your forties, you won't be able to get pregnant.
FACT: Irregular periods can go on for a couple of years before menopause actually occurs. That's why doctors recommend waiting for at least a year without any menstrual cycle before throwing away

your birth control pills—or any other forms of pregnancy prevention, for that matter.

Pregnancy

How it affects sexual response: Sexual response can be heightened during pregnancy because of increased blood flow and engorgement. The second trimester seems to be the most sexually satisfying for women. During the first three months of pregnancy breasts are especially tender and nausea is common. But during the second three months the queasiness has subsided and the hormones have caused an increase in vaginal lubrication. In the last three months most women are uncomfortable and not as easily sexually aroused. Some women are afraid to have intercourse at all while pregnant, for fear they will harm the baby, but in most cases with a healthy pregnancy, it's fine. Sexual intimacy is important during pregnancy as it keeps the couple emotionally and physically connected, which will benefit the unborn child. There are, however, some complications that indicate abstinence, such as bleeding, leakage of amniotic fluid, an incompetent cervix, or placenta previa, where the placenta lies low in the uterus. If the doctor recommends avoiding intercourse, kissing and hugging can keep the couple connected.

What to do: If having sex becomes uncomfortable or awkward as the abdomen continues to expand, varying and exploring different positions may be the answer. The ordinary missionary position can become difficult, but spooning, lying on the side, can work well. It is usually recommended to refrain from intercourse for six weeks following a vaginal or cesarean delivery. Women who have had an episiotomy, which is a surgical cut from the base of the vagina toward the anus to make it easier for the baby to come out, may need more time to heal before engaging in intercourse.

Women should also be aware of the possibility of postpartum depression, caused by the drastic change in hormone levels following the baby's birth. Women who have had depression in the past are particularly at risk, but no woman is immune. The symptoms range from depression, anxiety, and delusions to fears about hurting the baby. Women should be evaluated prior to their deliveries for risk factors for postpartum depression and seek help if the symptoms arise.

Pelvic-Floor Disorders

What it is: The pelvic floor is comprised of the muscles, ligaments, and fascia that support the pelvis. If any of these muscles or ligaments weaken or drop, they lose their supporting ability, which can lead to a prolapse of the bladder, uterus, or rectum. The prolapse can be the result of aging and menopause, a vaginal delivery that stretched the muscles, prior pelvic surgery such as a hysterectomy, or traumatic labor during childbirth. When a prolapse occurs, the bladder, uterus, rectum, and intestines can form a hernia in the wall of the vagina. Herniation of the bladder into the anterior wall of the vagina is a cystocele, the dropping of the rectum into the back wall of the vagina is a rectocele, and the bulging of the urethra is a urethracele. Prolapse of the uterus is when the uterus drops down into the vagina. Symptoms include a feeling of pressure in the vaginal area.

What to do: Kegel exercises can help strengthen the pelvic-floor muscles. Often vaginal physical therapy can help restore muscle tone and strength. For severe prolapse of the uterus or vagina, surgery may be required.

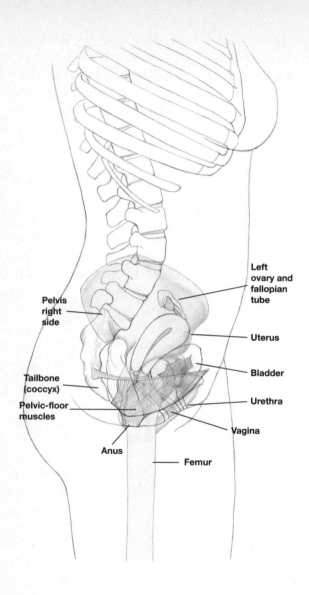

Pelvis right side

Tailbone (coccyx)

Pelvic-floor muscles

Anus

Left ovary and fallopian tube

Uterus

Bladder

Urethra

Vagina

Femur

Genital Pain

What it is: There are a number of reasons why a woman has genital pain. Some of the more common causes, which can also be associated with discomfort during intercourse, include:

- Fibroids (noncancerous growths in the uterus)
- Endometriosis (endometrial tissue that is normally found in the uterine lining that appears outside the uterus)
- Chronic pelvic inflammatory disease, or PID (long-term infections that cause fallopian tubes to scar)
- Vaginismus (involuntary muscle spasms of the lower third of the vagina, which can be caused by vaginal infections, sexually transmitted diseases, or ovarian cysts)
- Vulvodynia (chronic discomfort in the vulva without the presence of an infection)

University of Michigan researchers found that 27.9 percent of women have had pain in the vulva. In their web-based survey of 994 women, half of the respondents experienced pain during intercourse sometime in their life.

What to do: Treatment of any kind of genital pain depends on the cause. At our centers we have a comprehensive hormonal, topical, herbal, and physical therapy program for women with vaginal and pelvic pain. Sometimes nerve blocks are needed, and sometimes there is a nerve compression problem that can be relieved by injections and/or surgery.

STDs and HIV

What it is: Sexually transmitted diseases (STDs) are bacterial or viral infections that can be transferred from one person to another through sexual contact, which includes intercourse and oral, anal, and genital contact. Many times there are no symptoms and people are unaware that they have one. STDs can cause permanent bodily harm, and some sexually transmitted diseases can be passed to the fetus during pregnancy and birth. For many of the STDs, condoms offer the most protection. Bacterial STDs are curable with antibiotics, as long as treatment is not delayed. Viral STDs are incurable, although there is a vaccination available to prevent hepatitis B. Most STDs increase susceptibility to HIV infection.

Bacterial STDs include:

- **CHLAMYDIA.** Oftentimes there are no symptoms. It can cause an abnormal genital discharge, burning during urination, lower abdominal pain, vaginal bleeding, or painful intercourse. It can scar the fallopian tubes and affect a woman's ability to have children.
- **GONORRHEA.** It is characterized by a discharge from the vagina, pain, vaginal bleeding, and burning or itching during urination. If it goes untreated, it can cause sterility or pregnancy complications.
- **SYPHILIS.** There are different stages of the disease, and it begins with sores in the genitals or mouth. Next, a rash may appear, and in the late stage, it can cause brain or heart damage.

Viral STDs include:

- **GENITAL HERPES.** Caused by the herpes simplex virus (HSV), which is in the same family of viruses that cause chickenpox, shingles, and mononucleosis. There are two types of HSV: HSV-1, which appears on the lips in the form of cold sores, and HSV-2, which are lesions in the genital area. If someone has HSV-1 and performs oral sex, it is possible to give their partner genital herpes. It can lead to complications in pregnancy.
- **HUMAN PAPILLOMA VIRUS (HPV)** and genital warts can increase the risk of cervical cancer. A new test called HPV DNA can identify the virulent strains of HPV associated with cervical cancer.

- **HUMAN IMMUNODEFICIENCY VIRUS (HIV)** This virus weakens a person's immune system, causes flulike symptoms, and usually leads to severe illnesses and full-blown AIDS (acquired immune deficiency syndrome).

Obesity

Whether it is the result of too much fast food or a lack of exercise, obesity in America is on the rise. But obesity is not only a physical attraction issue, it's a health problem as well. Women who are overweight open themselves up to a host of medical problems, including diabetes, heart disease, hypertension, stroke, gallstones, menstrual irregularities, infertility, and problems with pregnancy. The Framingham Heart Study, reported in *The Annals of Internal Medicine,* found obesity to be associated with a decrease in life expectancy. The study involved 3,457 participants ages thirty to forty-nine at baseline. They concluded that forty-year-old female nonsmokers lost 3.3 years of their life because of being overweight. Obese female smokers lost 7.2 years compared with normal-weight smokers. Obese female smokers lost 13.3 years compared to normal-weight nonsmokers.

Doctors diagnose obesity by Body Mass Index (BMI), which is the measure of body fat based on height and weight. To figure your own BMI, multiply your weight in pounds by 705, divide that figure by your height in inches, then divide it by height in inches again. The formula is: BMI = (weight in pounds × 705) ÷ h (height in inches) ÷ h (height in inches). (There are also several websites that will calculate your BMI—all you have to do is type in your weight and height and they do the math.) People with a BMI greater than 25 are at an increased risk for heart problems.

Underweight = <18.5
Normal weight = 18.5–24.9

Overweight = 25–29.9

Obesity = 30 or greater

Other than overeating and lack of exercise, metabolic disorders, genetic makeup, and medications can cause weight gain and lead to obesity. Psychological components, too, can contribute to the problem. Overeating is often a way to fill some kind of empty emotional space inside. When someone feels depressed, afraid, or inadequate, food becomes a way to dull the pain and fill the void.

A person's weight has little to do with his or her ability to enjoy sex. Some of the most overweight women have the most satisfying sex lives. Still, many extremely heavy people don't feel attractive or sexy and stay away from sexual situations. They become self-conscious, say no to getting naked even when the lights are out, refuse to be touched by their partner, or evade sex altogether. Furthermore, high cholesterol levels that often go along with obesity can affect pelvic blood flow and sexual response.

Underweight

Women who are underweight may also steer clear of sexual situations. They may feel undesirable and/or have physical reasons why they don't have a sexual response. Their hormones may be altered because they have stopped menstruating as a result of an eating disorder. They may have a lack of libido or lack of genital sensation, both of which are related to the physiological changes associated with weighing too little. Being extremely thin can cause the same level of self-consciousness as being extremely heavy, and women who are underweight suffer from the same hormonal problems, such as low estrogen and dryness.

Kathy's Story

Kathy, age thirty-four, was thin yet had a body-image issue. She exercised incessantly and ate a very restrictive diet. She maintained such a low body weight that her estrogen levels dropped and for five years she didn't get a period. Her hormones became off-balance and she developed vaginal dryness, low energy, lack of sensation, and difficulty responding. Because of not getting her period she no longer felt feminine and became inhibited sexually. Finally, after almost a decade, she recovered from her eating disorder, started to gain weight, began menstruating again, and her reproductive system was back on track.

But putting weight back on was difficult for Kathy, especially since she had a distorted body image. Over time, and with the help of her supportive partner, she became accustomed to her new weight and her sex life improved.

GETTING YOUR SEX LIFE BACK ON TRACK

Resuming a normal sex life following a potentially life-threatening illness takes time and patience. No one battling a serious illness can expect his or her sex life to be normal immediately following treatment. Here are some ways to get back on track:

- Take it slow. Start off by cuddling, kissing, and touching.
- Accept the fact that you may have some difficulties resuming sex. Don't pressure yourself into having intercourse or achieving an orgasm right away.
- If any difficulty having sex continues for a lengthy period of time, consult your doctor. Don't be afraid to discuss it.

Sexual
Empowerment

We didn't concretely measure for sexual empowerment in our survey, but as you'll see, many of the characteristics of a sexually empowered woman were reflected in our sexually satisfied survey respondents. In our practices, we find that sexually satisfied women are sexually empowered. The results showed that women who enjoy life express themselves in the bedroom, have high self-esteem, know what arouses them, and are satisfied with their sex lives. We find that our patients who are content with their sex lives know what they want in the bedroom and how to go after it. They have an open mind, exude an air of self-confidence, and are in control—factors of both sexual satisfaction and sexual empowerment. A sense of sexual empowerment grows out of achieving communication in the bedroom,

FINDINGS FROM THE WOMEN'S SEXUAL SATISFACTION SURVEY

Sexually satisfied women say:

- They are pleased with how often they have sex.
- When having sex they are comfortable telling their partner what to do.
- They feel entitled to a fulfilling sex life.

relationship health, and everything else we have been discussing—it's the last stage of sexual satisfaction, when you have arrived!

Taking Charge:
Linda's Story

Linda was a married, forty-two-year-old social worker and mother of two. When she wasn't working she was cooking, carpooling, cleaning the house, and helping her kids with their homework. Her needs continuously took a backseat to those of her family. Although she would have sex with her husband regularly, she considered her love life to be regrettably mediocre. Then, when her son went off to college and her daughter entered high school, she vowed to turn her routine sex life around. With an empty nest just around the corner, she was eager to feel sensual, erotic, and enjoy lovemaking to the max.

In her twenty-two years of marriage Linda didn't resist sex, but she did not look forward to it either. She had occasional orgasms, but there was no pattern to when they occurred. She wasn't comfortable experimenting with different positions or exploring her body. All the while her husband was in the dark, unaware of her sexual dissatisfaction.

But before Linda could forge ahead, she needed to cast aside her hang-ups that affected intimacy. She needed to feel good about herself as a sexual partner and be receptive to receiving and giving pleasure. In other words, she needed to be "sexually empowered," which is essential in reaching your sexual peak. In therapy Linda was able to confront her insecurities, adopt skills to talk to her husband about what turned her on, and hold her own in a conflict resolution. After changing old habits, gaining overall confidence, and embracing her body, she was able to intensify her lovemaking. And, along with that, she became sexually empowered.

BUILDING A FOUNDATION

What is sexual empowerment—this state of being that puts you in charge of your sexual pleasure? What is this that can allow you to let down your guard and become more adventuresome between the sheets? To begin with, sexual empowerment interweaves all aspects of our lives—it's the way we feel about our genitalia as well as our physique. It's the way we see ourselves as individuals, as mothers, as wives and partners. It affects how we handle ourselves in relation to the outside world. While many women feel empowered in the workplace and in the gender role at home, they have difficulty embarking on or initiating erotic desires.

Although sexual empowerment and sexual satisfaction usually go hand in hand, they are not always the same. There may be a medical reason why you aren't sexually satisfied—you are experiencing a loss of desire because of stress, fatigue, the death of a loved one, anxiety, and depression. Relationship factors, too, such as unsolved conflicts with your partner, can squelch a once hot and heavy romance.

Below is a culmination of all the characteristics we have found that play a role in a sexually satisfied woman's sexual empowerment. Some of these have been explored in previous chapters, but in totality they represent a woman who has learned how to optimize and enjoy her sex life:

Having a good body image. Feeling good about the way you look. Even if you are having a bad hair day, are bloated from your period, and your jeans are too tight, you are still pretty proud of your body. You celebrate the way you look and feel and are content with your shape. You recognize you have imperfections and understand that everyone has flaws.

Feeling entitled to a fulfilling sex life. You recognize that you have a basic right to feel entitled to sexual pleasure. You are not too embarrassed or too uncomfortable to ask your partner for what you want.

Knowing what pleases you. You are not afraid to explore your body and learn to self-stimulate. You understand that you can't teach someone what arouses you unless you know firsthand.

Avoiding the use of drugs or alcohol as a crutch. You don't need any liquor or drugs to have fun in bed. This doesn't mean you can't enjoy a glass or two of wine, or have a drink before or after dinner. With or without addiction, some people can't become sexually involved without the use of mind-altering substances that help them relax. A sexually empowered person can loosen up, release inhibitions, and enjoy sex without the aid of drugs or alcohol.

Feeling confident about the number of sexual partners you have had. Whether you have had one, ten, or twenty sexual partners, you feel okay about it. Even if you wish you could forget a few of them, you can chalk it up to a case of bad judgment. You don't hide it if you have had several sexual partners, or feel pressured to lie about past experiences for fear your present partner will be turned off. If you are having sex for the right reasons and are enjoying an active sex life, and not using sex to find security or validation or attention, there is no reason to feel embarrassed. As long as you practice safe sex and do it for the right reasons, you believe there is nothing to hide.

Feeling comfortable about sexual orientation. Gay or straight, you are not hiding in the closet. Even though we have become more open as a society, there are still taboos against same-sex relationships. Being attracted to someone of the same sex can be shrouded in shame. It's not uncommon for anyone who is gay to be ostracized and judged by friends and family. Because of this, it is easy to internalize the negative messages concerning homosexuality. But being sexually empowered is being comfortable with whomever you are attracted to, male or female.

Maintaining an open mind. No matter what your sexual preference, you are accepting of other sexual lifestyles. People who are judgmental about homosexuality, for instance, may be uncomfortable with certain kinds of sexual activities and behaviors that may be thought of as lesbian, such as oral sex, role playing, fantasy, or watching different kinds of erotic movies. Females who feel homosexuality is sinful or dangerous or wrong are sometimes anxious about sex in general, but the open-minded, sexually empowered woman is open to sexual exploration.

Berman Footnote

Of all the experiences we have had in our life, most were not completely and purely homosexual or heterosexual. Think of yourself as on a continuum. It doesn't mean that if you have a (same-sex) fantasy, or if your partner acts out a homosexual fantasy, either one of you is homosexual. And if you are a homosexual woman and fantasize about having sex with a man, it doesn't mean you are heterosexual. It just means you are exploring different gender roles, which will enrich your sexual life. People who are more accepting of alternative lifestyles are

more accepting of experimentation in general, and that translates into a richer sex life.

CHANGING TIMES

Over the years attitudes toward women and sex have shifted, paving the way for empowerment. Because of the sexual revolution and the women's movement in the 1960s, great strides have been made. The barriers of gender expectation and gender stereotypes have opened up, and it is no longer presumed that the woman has to be the less dominant one in a relationship or in the workplace. The sexual revolution made it possible for women to enjoy sex openly and pursue it. The FDA's approval of the birth control pill alleviated the fear of unwanted pregnancy and changed the way many women felt about having sex. It sent the message that it was okay to enjoy sex without marriage or without the intention of having children. Still, women's liberation didn't automatically lead to empowerment.

Since the 1980s, sex has taken on a more negative element, with a realistic fear of AIDS, HIV, herpes, chlamydia, and the human papilloma virus, among other sexually transmitted diseases. Rightfully so, many women have refrained from multiple sex partners and have become prudent about practicing safe sex. But caution doesn't mean ceasing all passionate encounters.

Traditionally women have been made to feel uneasy and ashamed about placing an importance on their sex lives, and oftentimes women who did were considered promiscuous. At one time it was believed that women should just accept it when sex wasn't working, especially if they were over fifty. Now women are living longer and an active sex life is considered natural at any age. In our practice over the past several years, we have noticed that women have become more candid about their sexual appetites and are not afraid to seek help when physical problems, such as low libido, occur.

As women we get so many messages from an early age that can directly or indirectly repress our sexuality. In sex education in middle school and high school we learn how to protect ourselves from pregnancy, HIV, and sexually transmitted diseases. However, we get little to no instruction on how to achieve sexual pleasure. At home, it is highly unlikely that the topic of a family discussion at the dinner table is how to stimulate yourself. And on conventional television, sex chatters usually only address safe sex and risk factors.

Sexual empowerment is not something we are born with; rather, it's something that begins at an early age. Babies are born sexual. Studies have documented that babies will absentmindedly rub their genitals repeatedly against a teddy bear or a pillow, simply because it feels good. Children can reach orgasms very early in life, even though they don't ejaculate until puberty. Kids are aware of their sensory experiences and they know what feels good. It's how we grow into our sexuality that makes the difference.

The Power of Positive Thinking

A positive attitude toward sex is a central part of sexual empowerment. Consider these ways to lift your spirits—and a better sex life should soon follow:

Conquer negativity. Make a list of all the unfavorable messages you've received about your body and bodily functions growing up. Note which ones you still believe to be true, even though you may know intellectually they aren't. Once you make your list, try to turn these negative messages into positive ones that you can consistently refer to. For example, if the message is that good girls don't have sex until they're married, turn it around and tell yourself: "I'm not a bad person because I am unmarried and enjoy sex," or even better: "I'm a good person and I enjoy sex."

Focus on the positive. Your boyfriend broke up with you? Think of it as moving on to better fish in the sea. Think of it as a fresh start. Dwelling on a romance gone sour can prevent you from trusting again.

Add fun to your life. If you are overworked, bored, have no interest in sex, maybe it's because you are down in the dumps. Try adding some fun to your life. Go to the movies, see a play, visit a zoo, shop at a new boutique, explore a nearby city. This should be energizing, paving the way to rekindle the flames of passion.

Make a wish list. Write down ten things you would most like to do in life. Think of ways to make at least one of those wishes come true. Think of ten new ways to have fun in the bedroom. It doesn't have to be erotic positions for intercourse—it can be a full head-to-toe body massage from your partner.

MAN POWER

Men, more often than women, are raised with an automatic sense of sexual empowerment. They are encouraged from an early age to explore their sexuality. They get pats on the back when they have multiple sexual partners or when they have sex at all. This is not true for women, even today. If a woman has numerous sexual partners she is considered a slut. But each person has his or her own value system about how many sexual partners are acceptable.

The question is should women be more like men? Well, there are aspects of men's sexual empowerment that we can learn from. One feature of men's sexual lives is that they think about sex a lot. We are not trained or conditioned to think about sex all the time, and it doesn't even come naturally to us. But try thinking about sex more often. When you are walking down the street and see an attractive man, try to think about it for a split second. When sitting at your desk, do some Kegel exercises and think about your genitals for a minute. It doesn't mean that you are becoming sexually aroused. Men think about sex every three minutes. We won't achieve that statistic, but for women, thinking about sex more is a good start.

Women tend to be focused on the needs of others rather than on their own needs, as they take on more responsibility in life—a job, kids, a house. In order to think about sex, they have to turn everything else off and make a concerted effort; it probably won't come naturally. Yet women need to open up their minds to the sexual energy that's around them.

In trying to become more sexual, tune in to your body. Be aware of the different sensations in your genitals and try to think about it when you are watching a romantic movie, or reading a sex scene in your favorite romance novel. It's one way we can be more like men and feel more sexual in our daily lives. Women tend to compartmentalize their lives—when they are being a mother, they are just a mother; when they are working, they are just at work—and it's the same when they are having sex. But women need to stop separating their different roles. Incorporating sex into your life doesn't mean engaging in sex twenty-four hours a day—it just means incorporating a sense of sexuality.

TIME OUT

To be sexually empowered you need to set time aside for yourself. Most women strive to be super-functional nurturers and rarely make themselves a priority. A large part of their self-concept and self-esteem comes from nurturing and caring for others. It is considered self-indulgent at worst, irresponsible at best, when a woman puts aside her other "responsibilities" to take care of herself beyond the basics, such as going to the doctor or dentist, or getting her hair cut. But if we don't take care of ourselves physically, emotionally, and spiritually there is no room for sexual energy toward our relationships. This is common in today's modern woman who spends the whole day caring for children, working, or some combination thereof. It's hard to be empowered if all your energy is focused on taking care of others.

In an effort to focus on your own needs, try to do the following:

Please yourself. Take notice of your nurturing behavior and think about ways you can please yourself. Maybe it's with regular exercise, or a standing manicure appointment, or a weekly lunch date with friends.

Be creative. Make a wish list of ways to pamper yourself. Perhaps it's a class you've been longing to take, a routine you'd like to start, or a trip you want to take.

Stop making excuses. You don't have to be perfect when taking care of others. It's okay to go partway instead of 100 percent each time. Laura recently met a woman who was on a journey of self-nurturance. She told her that she had been avoiding taking a pottery class because she couldn't imagine devoting the time it would require to be good at it, such as time at the studio, hours on weekends, and classes every week. When asked why she wanted to do pottery she said it was something she had always dreamed about, and that she loved the idea of working with the earth and the meditative quality of operating the wheel. Through their exploration she realized that she didn't have to be a master ceramics artist to gain the benefits, and that no one would judge her if she wasn't perfect. Sometimes it's important to start a new activity or routine one step at a time, setting realistic expectations.

Mommy's Private Time:
Sophia's Story

When Sophia was thirty-eight she was bogged down with her three small children. She had put her career as a lawyer on hold and devoted all her time to carting her kids around to soccer practice, ballet lessons, art classes, and story time at the local library. When her husband, Kevin, came home from work, she was exhausted, and her yearning for loving was at an all-time low. Kevin, frustrated that their sex life was almost nonexistent, suggested Sophia hire a sitter two afternoons a week so she could have some alone time. Sophia made a list of things she wanted to do but never got around to, and one by one, thanks to the sitter, she was able to accomplish them. One time it was meeting an old friend for lunch, another time it was an afternoon at the spa, and one afternoon she simply stayed in her bedroom with the door shut and read a book or watched a movie on cable TV. By giving herself permission to have some private time without the children, she felt renewed and ready for fun in bed.

TUNING IN TO YOUR SENSUALITY

Spending time focusing on your sensuality is another way to nurture yourself. Laura often uses exercises and suggestions from Bernard Gunther's *Sense* and Patrick Carnes's *Sexual Anorexia* with patients who are trying to reconnect to their sensuality. Here is our version of what they suggest:

Cleanse in slow motion. Try a new, deliberately slow way to wash yourself. Test the water until it's warm, then close your eyes and leisurely and generously lather up. Tune in to the sensation of the soapy suds touching your skin. Spread the foamy soap all over your face, arms, hands, and neck. Cup the soothing water into your hands and splash your face. Concentrate on how you rinse. Pick up a soft towel and gently press it against your face. Focus on how the terry-cloth feels against your skin. Pat your skin dry.

Attention, please. Close your eyes and listen to the sounds of the room. Feel your breath, listen to your heartbeat, and notice the room's temperature on your face and body. Become aware of how your clothes meet your skin. Feel the way your feet press against the carpet or floor.

Bend and stretch. Close your eyes and lie flat on your back on the floor. Concentrate on how your body feels resting on the ground. Without straining, stretch each part of your body. Start with your toes and move up to your head. Notice which muscle groups feel good to stretch, and which ones are painful when extended.

Savor an orange. Place an orange in the palm of your hand. Smell and feel the peel. Examine the texture and hues. With your eyes closed, roll the orange in your hands, up and down your forearms, across your face, shoulders, and neck. Slowly remove the peel, sniffing the aroma and feeling the juice squirt on your skin. Separate the sections, keeping your eyes closed. Put a small section in your mouth, lick it, feel it against your mouth, take a bite, feeling the juice on your tongue. Repeat this with each section of the orange.

Silence is golden. Dine in silence. Eat a three- or four-course meal with a friend, relative, or partner—without saying a word. Maintain eye contact with your dinner partner while you are chewing and swallowing. Periodically close your eyes.

Composition 101. Write a sensual and/or sexual fantasy. Make it erotic and sensational, and include information about your senses. If your fantasy takes place on a beach, describe the sounds of the sea, the taste of the saltwater, and the feeling of the grainy sand on your toes and hands. Picture yourself making love on a deserted stretch of the shoreline. Share your fantasies and sensations with your partner.

The eyes of the beholder. For the next month concentrate on what you find erotic about your partner, and don't limit it to the blatantly sexual. Look for small things, like the curve of a neck, his or her hair, a smile, a particular look, etcetera. Write them down as you notice them and share your thoughts.

TEST YOURSELF

Do you think you have what it takes to be sexually empowered? Take this quiz to see how sexually empowered you really are. Answer "yes" to the statements you would agree with.

1.	I think positively about my sexuality several times a day.	yes	no
2.	I feel like I'm a good lover, or at least I have the capacity to be.	yes	no
3.	I'm comfortable telling my partner what I want during sex.	yes	no
4.	I communicate my sexual desires as often as I wish.	yes	no
5.	I'm motivated to avoid engaging in "risky" (e.g., unprotected) sexual behavior.	yes	no
6.	I feel comfortable initiating sexual activity with my partner.	yes	no
7.	My sexuality is something I feel responsible for.	yes	no
8.	I'm proud of the way I deal with and handle my sexual desires and needs.	yes	no
9.	I have the skills and ability to ensure rewarding sexual behaviors for myself.	yes	no

10. I know all the parts of my sexual anatomy and
    how they work.   yes no

11. I feel comfortable being nude with a partner.   yes no

SCORING:

If you answered yes to:

0–4 OUT OF THE 11 ITEMS: Take a close look at your no answers, as
these issues may be playing a negative role in your sexual health.

6–8 OUT OF THE 11 ITEMS: You have some strengths and in certain
areas may feel sexually empowered, but there are areas where you
are still struggling. You may want to try to build up your levels of
confidence in those areas where you replied no.

9–11 OUT OF 11 ITEMS: You want to pay attention to anything you
are lacking, but you are on the right track. Even if you say yes to all of
the above, and are on the higher end of sexual empowerment, there
is always room for improvement.

BOTTOM LINE

There is no reason why your sex life has to fall short. Once all your
ducks are in order—you have honed your communication skills, worked
on your romance, taken control of your mental health, dealt with your
past, attended to your physical health, and believed wholeheartedly that
you are entitled to good sex—you are on the road to sexual empowerment. You may face stumbling blocks along the way, it's to be expected, but they can be overcome. Once you have gotten to the point
where you can say you are sexually empowered, you are not far away
from achieving sexual satisfaction.

Attitudes and Sex Across the Generations

This chapter is about attitudes toward sex. In our study we found that sexual attitudes were not significantly related to sexual satisfaction. We asked respondents how they felt about the importance of a satisfying sex life, premarital sex, gay relationships, sex without love, teen sex, and infidelity. And their answers leaned toward the conservative side. However, in our practice, we find that as a general

---

FINDINGS FROM THE WOMEN'S SEXUAL SATISFACTION SURVEY

The biggest differences between generations were their views on:

- Premarital sex
- Alternative lifestyles
- Multiple sex partners
- Oral sex

---

rule older adults tend to be less permissive and younger adults tend to be more liberal than the generations before them.

Although there are no consistent attitudes defining the sexually satisfied woman, a look at sexual attitudes across generations can be helpful in understanding sexual satisfaction. Knowing how sexual views have changed from our mothers' and grandmothers' time gives us an insight into what sexual satisfaction has come to mean.

An Awakening:
A Grandmother's Story

When Amy was age twelve and her brother Seth was nine they went on a family vacation with their mother, father, and grandmother. Their parents came of age sexually in the 1960s, the beginning of the sexual revolution, and they raised Amy and Seth to be open about sex. Their grandmother, though, came of sexual age in the late 1930s, before World War II, and sex in her household was never mentioned above a whisper, if at all.

Within a few days of sitting in the car with Amy and Seth, their grandmother had an awakening. Sex and raw language were a part of the backseat conversation. She was quite surprised at the dialogue. "We sure didn't talk like that in front of our parents in my day," she had said. By the end of the trip the natural sex talk was no longer noteworthy.

There is no doubt that there are differences between generations that can and do affect our attitudes and our sexuality.

ATTITUDES

Social norms, religious beliefs, parental influences, and peer pressure can all influence one's attitudes. Here is what sexually satisfied women in the survey feel about the following four issues:

Teen Sex

What they say: Teenagers are not mature enough to have sex.

Bottom line: Like it or not, for generations teenagers have been having sex. Unfortunately, getting pregnant, risking STDs and HIV and AIDS, and being rejected afterward are realities. For parents, teen sex is a frightening thought. According to the National Campaign to Prevent Teen Pregnancy, almost half (46 percent) of high school teens in the United States have had sexual intercourse. The *New York Times Magazine* cover story on May 30, 2004, addressed the issue of casual sex being on the rise among teenagers. They found that of the 55 percent of eleventh graders who engaged in intercourse, 60 percent said they had sex with a friend rather than a partner in a relationship. The article pointed out that "friends with benefits" allows the kids to release sexual tensions without an emotional attachment or worrying about getting hurt. The survey had been conducted by Bowling Green

State University in Ohio. The article also reported that oral sex is common among eighth and ninth graders. Many teenagers are replacing intercourse with oral sex. Kids have been inundated with information about intercourse and AIDS, and believe that oral sex is safer. But in fact, oral sex is not risk-free. They are not as educated about the potential consequences of oral sex.

Finding privacy and opportunities for sex is easier than ever for today's teenager. Cell phones and the Internet are changing the way teens date. They can now privatize their lives without their parents' knowledge. Before kids had their own cell phones, they received calls at home, often with their parents answering the call. But with e-mail and cell phones, parents are unaware who is calling, when, or why.

Berman Footnote .

Sex comes with a large degree of responsibility, and teenagers should work within their family's value system and not have sex until they are ready to face the emotional and physical consequences, such as becoming pregnant, getting STDs, or being rejected afterward. Becoming sexually active shouldn't happen until someone has the emotional security to cope with the potential consequences. The fun part of sex is easy, but the potential consequences can be devastating.

How do you know when you are ready to have sex?

- When you have a birth control plan in place
- When you understand safe-sex practices and how to use them
- When you are able to negotiate safe-sex practices with a partner who may not be as willing

It's been estimated that the first sexual experience for 80 percent of teenagers wasn't a positive one—they don't consider themselves to have been forced, but see themselves as just giving in to the pressure from their partner, or just to be part of the crowd. But having a negative first sexual experience can have an impact on the rest of your sexual life because it is at a key point in your development. It can kick-start your sexual life in a negative way.

Sex without Marriage

What they say: Without that wedding ring on your finger, think twice before having intercourse.

Bottom line: Millions of American women choose to have sex before they marry. A couple of generations ago, sleeping with your partner before you walked down the aisle may have raised many eyebrows. According to *Sex in America: A Definitive Survey* (see Appendix), of those women born between 1933 and 1942, 90 percent were either virgins when they married or had premarital intercourse only with the man they married. While premarital sex was once unusual, today it's commonplace. The social taboos have been lifted, there isn't the same stigma, and people aren't judged to the same degree.

> 38.6 percent of respondents thought sex before marriage was not wrong at all.
> 25.4 percent thought it was wrong sometimes.
> 36.1 percent thought it was almost always, or always, wrong.

Another reason why sex before marriage is more prevalent is that women are getting married later. Many couples live together before they marry, date for a long time, remain single and experiment with a lot of sexual partners. Still, some religions frown upon premarital sex, and consider it a sin. The belief is that virginity is a virtue. Some women feel it's a part of their value system and would feel guilty having intercourse before saying their "I do's."

The decision is very individual. Here are some pros and cons of having sexual intercourse before marriage:

Pros. If you have intercourse before marriage, you are able to work on your sexual communication and determine if there are any sexual conflicts before making that commitment. Although most often difficulties can be worked through, discovering your partner has a sexual preference or fetish that is incompatible with your beliefs or needs can be frightening. It doesn't mean that if you wait until your wedding night to have sex that your marriage will be doomed. But if you have sex before marriage, your wedding night and the beginning of your relationship will not be marred by any major surprises.

Cons. Many people find the waiting exciting. If someone is abstaining because of moral or religious beliefs, then if they have sex before marriage they will feel guilty and not enjoy it. If your partner is also a virgin, then you can share the "first time" experience together.

For women who believe sex before marriage is wrong, a marriage license may not be enough to suddenly turn on the light switch of passion. If they spent their whole lives repressing a part of their sexuality and believing their sexual instincts and desires are dangerous, it can be hard to embrace them when finally given the permission to be sexual.

Christine and Justin's Story

Christine and Justin were twenty-six years old when they got married and both waited to have intercourse until their wedding night. As a result, they had a lot of problems getting started in their sexual relationship. Neither one knew what to do or understood their body. In trying to remain virgins, they kept their sexual feelings at bay. Then, when they found themselves husband and wife, they had a hard time opening up sexually. Not only did they still have the guilt they had carried around with them, but they also were embarrassed about sex and found it awkward to feel sensual. They needed to do a lot of work building their sex life from the bottom up, starting with giving themselves permission to be sexual and learning how to communicate their sexual needs. Eventually they developed a fulfilling sex life, but it took a long time.

Christine and Justin weren't sorry they waited until they took their wedding vows to have intercourse, as it was a part of their religious value system, but they were surprised how hard it was. They had always believed that as soon as they married it would be so wonderful, but for them it wasn't a great experience.

No Love, No Sex

> 83 percent of respondents thought you shouldn't have sex without love.

What they say: Sex should only occur with love.

Bottom line: Is this a surprise? Not at all. For most of us, sex is much more than physical release. It's the emotional bond, intimacy, and love that make sex satisfying. Unrequited love is also not rewarding. Instead, when love is one-sided, it's heartbreaking. When most women fantasize about being in love it's mutual, but unfortunately it doesn't always work that way. You may be in love but your partner may not, and when there is a physical relationship the rejection can be devastating. Some women engage in sex as a way to keep their partner. They fear their partner will have sex with someone else if they don't, or leave them if they are not giving themselves completely.

Laura hears countless stories about women who sleep with their partners to keep them, only to be jilted anyway. If a person really cares about you, he (or she) shouldn't be pressuring you to have sex. Having sex to keep your partner is more common among younger women. We see this with adolescents. They feel deeply in love with their partner and there is an inherent unspoken or spoken expectation that if they don't have sex that partner will leave them for someone who will.

The Unwanted Birthday Present: David's Story

David was still in high school when he came to see Laura for advice after a sex education class. His sixteen-year-old girlfriend, Abby, wanted to give him her virginity as a birthday present, but he wasn't sure if he should accept. David was very fond of Abby, but he wasn't madly in love. He was young, had the rest of high school and college ahead of him, and just about the last thing he wanted to do was make a long-term commitment. Laura and David talked about the ramifications of being Abby's first lover. Although Abby said giving herself to him was a symbol of her love, he wasn't comfortable accepting that responsibility. David did some soul-searching and decided that accepting her offer would be setting her up to be hurt. Although he cared a great deal for her, he knew that he didn't love her the way she claimed to love him, and eventually the relationship would end. The inevitable rejection, no matter when it occurred, would set up a negative cycle for her sexual life and she would associate sex with rejection, a sense of loss and humiliation. David unselfishly turned down her offer, in the best interest of Abby.

Younger girls tend to be more impulsive than older girls. They may be more easily pressured into sex, and quicker to jump into bed with a partner without thinking through motivations and consequences. While older women may have the same kinds of strong feelings as younger women, they have more realistic expectations. Just from life experiences alone, older women will likely understand that engaging in sex doesn't assume the relationship will have longevity. Still, when older women develop an emotional attachment after establishing a sexual relationship, they, too, are open to being hurt.

Some women can successfully have sex buddies with whom they have a physical relationship and no emotional attachment. But what often happens is that when they do begin to have sex on a regular basis, emotions develop, complicating the situation.

Pornography

13.3 percent of respondents bought or rented an X-rated movie in the past year.

What they say: Most wouldn't rent an X-rated movie or read what they considered pornography.

Bottom line: Pornographic magazines and X-rated movies are designed to inspire and maintain fantasy. A lot of couples find that watching X-rated movies or reading erotic magazines can help to spice up their sex life. It gets them in the mood, gives them ideas of things to try. They can watch together and express what they like and what they don't. As we mentioned, with Internet access, couples can order X-rated films online from the comfort of their own home instead of physically visiting shops they may find intimidating or embarrassing. Men, in particular, enjoy them and it's an experience you may want to share with your partner. There are female-friendly erotica geared for women, which means they have a plot and the women in the films are not being sexually humiliated, and in many cases, are sexually empowered. Female-friendly films don't represent women in a humiliating fashion and are often softer in nature, with a plot women can relate to.

Only 6 percent of respondents bought a sexually explicit magazine or book within the past year. Only .8 percent paid by the minute for phone sex.

BACK IN TIME

In the process of exploring sexual satisfaction, we wanted to look at the data, compare the different age groups, and see what role culture played in their sexual attitudes. Which groups were similar? Which social environments were more conducive to liberal views? Which ones have more conservative thinking? We divided age into four categories:

GROUP: The Ozzie and Harriets
AGE: Over 60 (12 percent)
These women were born in the 1940s or earlier, and came into their sexuality around the 1950s.

GROUP: The Free Lovers
AGE: 46–60 (31 percent)
These women were born in the 1940s and 1950s and came of age in the 1960s.

GROUP: The Disco Divas
AGE: 31–45 (43 percent)
These women were born around the 1960s and 1970s and began their sexual years in the 1970s and 1980s.

GROUP: The Generation X'ers
AGE: 18–30 (23 percent)
These women were born in the 1970s and 1980s and became sexual in the 1980s and 1990s.

In order to understand and explore each generation of women, it's helpful to take a look at the political, social, and sexual climate of each decade. Each generation was exposed to events, crises, pop culture trends, and political correctness that shaped their beliefs and attitudes during their sexual development. Here is a summary highlighting the 1950s, 1960s, 1970s, and 1980s.

The 1950s (The Ozzie and Harriets)

Eisenhower was in office (1953–1961), Senator Joseph McCarthy was targeting alleged communists in the United States, Dr. Jonas Salk developed a vaccine for polio, and Rosa Parks refused to go to the back of the bus in Alabama. The Supreme Court desegregated schools in *Brown vs. the Board of Education* and Julius and Ethel Rosenberg were electrocuted for treason. Elvis Presley became the king of rock 'n' roll and Buddy Holly and the Big Bopper were killed in a plane crash. *I Love Lucy, Ozzie and Harriet*, and *The Honeymooners* had families glued to their TVs, and *Gentlemen Prefer Blondes* hit the big screen, making Marilyn Monroe a movie star sex symbol and icon. Dick Clark's *American Bandstand* was the reality TV of the fifties, and brought music to the big tube. Little girls played with baby dolls, boys sported toy guns and cowboy gear, and both sexes twirled their hula hoops. In 1959, the Barbie doll was introduced at the American International Toy Fair in New York. Poodle skirts, petticoats, and penny loafers were fashionable garb. Betty Crocker's cookbook was the domestic goddess's bible. Drive-in movies became a sexy date destination. The Kinsey Report came out reporting on sexual mores and practices in the United States. An after-school activity for girls was charm school, where they were taught the proper way to walk and talk, dinner table etiquette, and dating protocol.

Women who came of age in the fifties were on the tail end of World War II and raised with very traditional gender roles and traditional expectations. Women were taught that they should have sex only in the confines of marriage. It was before birth control was readily available. Women were encouraged to lie back and satisfy their husbands. Their primary goal was to be emotionally and sexually a good wife to their spouses.

The 1960s (The Free Lovers)

John F. Kennedy became president of the United States, beating Richard M. Nixon. Martin Luther King Jr. gave his "I had a dream" speech. President Kennedy was assassinated in Dallas, Texas, on November 22, 1963, and Lee Harvey Oswald, the accused killer, was shot by Jack Ruby. Lyndon B. Johnson became the country's new president, and two years later he increased our involvement in Vietnam. Sit-ins and protests became commonplace, especially on college campuses. In 1968, King was assassinated and two months later Robert Kennedy, JFK's brother, died at the hands of an assassin. In 1969, Neil Armstrong and Buzz Aldrin were the first Americans to walk on the moon. Long hair, miniskirts, hot pants, and Mod clothes were the latest fashion. Heavily sprayed bouffants and flips were the "must have" hairstyles. The British rock stars the Beatles took the country by storm and Beatlemania reigned. Woodstock was the weekend of music, love, and sex for a half million youngsters. Bob Dylan and Peter, Paul and Mary were putting messages to music. The rock musical *Hair* opened Off-Broadway in 1967, soon moving to Broadway, and nudity and antiestablishment themes hit the stage. People were tuning into *Bewitched, Gunsmoke*, and *I Dream of Jeannie* on the small screen. Betty Friedan published *The Feminine Mystique* and the Food and Drug Administration approved the birth control pill.

With the availability of the pill, "free love" became common practice; it was acceptable, and sometimes even encouraged, to have multiple partners and explore your sexuality. Sex and pregnancy were now separated as concepts, so sex could be as much for fun as for procreation. There still wasn't much focus on orgasm or what to do with low desire; the tone of the time was much more about sexual exploration for women rather than sexual satisfaction.

The 1970s (The Disco Divas)

Richard Nixon was reelected president only to be disgraced because of the Watergate scandal and forced to resign. Gerald Ford became president, then Jimmy Carter won the election in 1978. Patty Hearst was kidnapped, and the Jim Jones religious cult mass suicide left more than nine hundred dead at Jonestown, Guyana. Fashionistas wore platform shoes and bell-bottom jeans. *Star Wars* hit the big screen and *All in the Family* and *The Mary Tyler Moore Show* were cutting-edge television sitcoms. Disco dancing, *Saturday Night Fever*, and heavy metal music topped the pop culture's latest craze. *Ms.* magazine was founded, and in 1973 the landmark decision *Roe v. Wade* gave women a constitutional right to have an abortion.

There was more focus on sexual pleasure for women than ever before, and sex therapy was becoming much more available. Books like *My Secret Garden* by Nancy Friday and *The Joy of Sex* by Alex Comfort were just a few of the sexual resources published during this time that set the stage for the beginnings of sexual empowerment for women. Consciousness-raising groups not only addressed social advocacy and professional and social empowerment, but many groups led by sex therapists focused on helping women achieve sexual pleasure. The practice of swinging and sex with multiple partners was at an all-time high, and women were becoming much less intimidated about initiating sex. These Disco Divas were raised by the Ozzie and Harriets, moving well beyond their mothers' value systems while challenging them. There was often friction between mothers and daughters due to the extreme difference in attitudes toward gender roles and sexuality.

The 1980s (The Generation X'ers)

Ronald Reagan was elected president, defeating Jimmy Carter; Pan Am Flight 103 exploded over Lockerbie, Scotland, and Libyan terrorists claimed responsibility for the bomb. The Berlin Wall came dow

John Lennon was assassinated, and the space shuttle *Challenger* exploded. Tampons were associated with toxic shock syndrome, Prozac was introduced as an antidepressant, French scientist Dr. Luc Montagnier discovered HIV, the virus that causes AIDS. Sally Ride became the first woman in space. Cabbage Patch dolls became a must for little girls, *The Cosby Show* was a TV hit and *Dallas* became a nighttime soap opera ratings buster. Condom commercials started to air on the small screen. Torn jeans, tank tops, and sneakers were the coveted casual garb.

This began the era of HIV and AIDS, which brought a lot of negative messages and fear around sex. Sex became associated with death. Girls coming of age sexually in the 1980s were raised by the Free Lovers who spearheaded the women's movement. Although these girls were exposed to open sexual ideals, they had limitations as sex became associated with scary consequences. Sexual experimentation was off the table for a while. Unlike the Free Lovers and Disco Divas, these women were now back to condom use and struggling with how to negotiate for safer sex.

TIMES THEY ARE A-CHANGING: AN OVERVIEW

The most conservative group, the women over sixty, were the least likely to have premarital sex or partake in unconventional sexual behavior. For these women, the image of the ideal was Doris Day, good girl, virginal, and pure love. Only "tramps" slept around. Being raised in a pre–birth control era, they were much more cautious and concerned about getting pregnant. Having a baby "out of wedlock" was a disgrace.

The Ozzie and Harriets' children were the Disco Divas. Unlike their parents, the Disco Divas cohabitated with their boyfriends, something almost unheard of with the older generations. This created conflicts between parents and children, with anger and distance developing.

The Free Lovers, the forty-six- to sixty-year-olds, were much more liberal than the previous group. With the advent of the pill, sexual behavior and attitudes took a big turn. Women no longer had to wait to have sex, and premarital sexual relations became acceptable. Although the pill alleviated some of the fear of getting pregnant before marriage, the idea of having a baby out of wedlock still carried with it shame and a stigma.

The Free Lovers came of age during the sexual revolution and were much more vocal and proactive about changing the world. Their attitudes and behaviors were a drastic change from that of their parents. They began to explore and experiment with their sexuality. They were not ashamed to seek out X-rated magazines and videos when they became available. These are the baby boomers, and their children are the Generation X'ers. They raised children who felt entitled to social equality and social change. These women as well as their children benefited from a new level of sexual empowerment. It was much more normal for girls to grow up expecting sexual satisfaction.

The Disco Divas expanded upon the attitudes of the Free Lovers and took them to the next level by adding a brand of feminism and empowerment. Instead of flower power and nature, these women were assertive and overtly sexual, spending time on the club scene and exploring their social and sexual power. In many ways their attitudes toward free love were not much different from the generation before them, but the social empowerment added another dimension to being an openly sexual woman.

With the AIDS scare, the Generation X'ers, instead of continuing on the upswing of free love, were suddenly faced with serious consequences related to sex. Sexual freedom leveled off as sexual exploration became associated with fear and stigma. This generation refrained from certain sexual experimentation and behaviors. Although they were not as conservative as the over-sixty group, they were much more uptight about having multiple partners than t[...] Disco Divas and Free Lovers before them.

Eventually some of the myths of AIDS were dispelled, such [...] agnosis automatically means a death sentence, women with [...]

have children, it can be transferred by kissing and you can contract it by ordinary contact. This would account for the upsurge of liberalism toward sex by some of the younger Generation X'ers. These women were the most open-minded in their sexual attitudes and behavior, and felt the most comfortable expressing their sexual needs.

It is interesting that the two middle groups—the thirty-one- to forty-five- and the forty-six- to sixty-year-olds—had very little difference in their attitudes. One came of age in the sixties and one in the seventies and they weren't drastically different environments. The big difference was found between the youngest and the oldest groups.

OUR SURVEY FINDINGS

Sexual Satisfaction

Age wasn't relevant to sexual satisfaction. It may have to do with the balance between sexual expectations and sexual assertiveness. For example, women in the fifties didn't have access to the information we have today about sexual health. No one talked about it, and their expectations for sex were more about the needs of their partners than anything else. They have carried these expectations with them throughout the years. However, younger women are much more accustomed than their grandmothers to accessing the extensive resources and information available to them, and have been raised to have much higher standards for what they expect out of sex. They are much more comfortable and adept at advocating for themselves. So perhaps the reason there appears to be no difference in sexual satisfaction among different age groups is because each generation of women has their own balance between their expectations and their willingness to advocate for their sexual needs and feel fulfilled.

Sexual Attitudes

- **The Generation X'ers had more liberal sexual attitudes overall than other age groups, and the Ozzie and Harriets had the most conservative attitudes. Women in the two middle-age categories (Free Lovers and Disco Divas) did not differ from each other on sexual attitudes.**

As we have said, the Ozzie and Harriets had many more restrictions placed on their sexuality and sexual development, given the climate in which they were raised. There was a stigma about having sex, or certainly a baby, before marriage; there wasn't access to information or a birth control pill. The Generation X'ers had the most access to information and education about sex and the biggest exposure to sex in the media, as explicit sex on the big screen became more prevalent. They also have the advantage of many new and evolving innovations in birth control, such as Ortho Evra, the birth control patch that women can wear a week at a time. There is also NuvaRing, a hormone-impregnated silicone ring a woman inserts in her vagina for three weeks; she then takes it out for a week and gets her period. The FDA approved a new birth control pill in 2003 called Seasonale that is taken continuously for three-month periods at a time, allowing a woman to menstruate only four times a year.

- **The Generation X'ers perceived that they were more attractive than women in the other age groups.**

With a focus on youth and beauty in our culture, it's not surprising that the youngest generation perceives itself as more attractive. This generation has gotten the message through movies, TV commercials, and fashion that the younger you are, the more beautiful you are. This is reinforced by men who appear to be more attracted to young, trimmer, physically firmer, and wrinkle-free women.

This generation is also more physically fit than the older

tions. When women over sixty grew up, going to the gym wasn't even in their vocabulary. Today many eighteen- to thirty-year-olds are diligent, even obsessed, about working out and eating right.

Sexual Behavior

- Women age forty-six and older were least likely to buy any sex-related materials, and engage in various kinds of sexual behaviors including oral and anal sex. The Generation X'ers were more likely to do both.

Once again, the permissive sexual climate and availability of resources over the Internet may have led to easy access and lack of taboos for this youngest generation of women.

- The Generation X'ers reported that they had a better sex life in the past twelve months than did women in the other age groups. The Generation X'ers and Disco Divas were the most likely to have had a sexual partner in the last twelve months, but the X'ers were the most likely to have multiple partners. The Ozzie and Harriets reported that they had the worst sex life in the past twelve months compared to women in any other age group, and were the least likely to have multiple sex partners let alone even one partner.

The younger women probably reported better sex lives because of the availability of partners, fewer responsibilities, and less sexual dysfunction than women in the older groups. Many Generation X'ers are in college, or enjoying single life, perhaps with a steady boyfriend. Odds are the Disco Divas are married or engaged, accounting for the likelihood of a partner. As a woman ages, especially when she reaches sixty and beyond, she is more apt to have a spouse pass away than the younger women and to experience physiological changes that inter-fere with sex.

- The Generation X'ers and Disco Divas were more likely to "always" perform and receive oral sex. The two older groups, the Free Lovers and Ozzie and Harriets, were least likely. These two groups were also more likely to say they never masturbated in the past year.

The openness and willingness to engage in oral sex may have as much to do with available partners, discussed above, as the difference in conservatism of sexual attitudes between generations. Women over sixty have physiological, hormonal, and genital blood flow changes that may impact on sexual desire and energy, preventing the inspiration to masturbate. Furthermore, they grew up in a generation where there was no education and information about masturbation and they were already well into their sexual years by the time that information was becoming commonplace in women's conversations. Unless they had a younger daughter who clued them in, or they educated themselves, they wouldn't have the information they need to explore self-stimulation.

Intimacy, Communication

- The Generation X'ers were more likely to use both words and touching to communicate their sexual needs to their partner, and Ozzie and Harriets were the least likely. The X'ers were more likely to say that intimacy with their partner was "excellent" compared to other women. Women over forty-six were less likely to say intimacy was "excellent" compared to other women.

The women more apt to communicate were those who are empowered, were raised by the baby boomers, and able to advocate for their sexual and emotional needs. They also socialize with a generation open-minded and emotionally available men raised by the same eration of Free Love and Disco Diva mothers, who encourage ble gender roles and the ability to effectively communicate their feelings. These younger women had the vocabulary, and both the social and maternal permission, to feel entitled to speak up for their sexual needs, more so than prior generations. They also have models in the media, and more of a sense of permission.

Sexual Dysfunction

- The Ozzie and Harriets reported they would feel the worst, compared to other women in the sample, if they were to spend the rest of their life with the same level of sexual functioning they have now. They had more urinary tract problems and said that their sex life was negatively affected by vaginal dryness. The Generation X'ers seemed to feel better than the other generations about the possibility of staying with their same level of sexual function. They also had fewer urinary problems and were least affected by vaginal dryness.

  Women over sixty don't want to spend their life at their present level of sexual function because of factors related to age resulting in decreased sexual response and pleasure. It is expected that with lower estrogen and testosterone levels and lower genital blood flow, this group of women would be struggling with lower libido, vaginal dryness, and vaginal atrophy. They had more urinary problems because, with age, bladder difficulties increase due to changes in hormonal status and childbirth, which can eventually lead to urinary incontinence.

- The Generation X'ers were less likely to be on antidepressants (11 percent) than were Disco Divas (17 percent), Free Lovers (21 percent), or Ozzie and Harriets (18 percent).

  The highest incidence of women who were on antidepressants were the Free Lovers. These are the women going through perimenopause and menopause. It could be these women are experiencing mood changes related to hormonal fluctuations, empty nest issues, social changes, and pressures of raising teenagers, all of which may put them at risk for a higher incidence of depression.

Berman Footnote About Mother/Daughter Relationships

Each generation of daughters is swayed by their mothers. But it works both ways. Kids can also influence their parents by challenging their comfort level and belief systems, pushing the envelope. For some mothers it can lead to reevaluating their own values. In many relationships it brings the parents and children closer together.

In keeping an open mind, mothers and daughters can learn from each other. The daughter can learn from her mother's life experiences, and the mother can learn about life from her daughter's perspective. Both can see situations in an altogether different light. It doesn't mean that either one has to adopt the other's values, but they can both open their eyes to a different point of view.

Pivotal Influences

Over the past decades there have been many pivotal factors that have changed our sexual thinking and behavior, helping to get us where we are today. While the list of what helped to empower women is endless, here are some of the significant influences that we have encountered:

- ACCEPTANCE OF HOMOSEXUALITY. Until the 1970s homosexual acts were illegal and psychiatrists considered homosexuality an emotional problem that had to be cured. In 1973, the American Psychiatric Association determined that homosexuality was no longer considered a mental illness. Alternative lifestyles gradua' became more acceptable. This is not to say that there isn't st' stigma related to homosexuality. Some religions still consider it a sin, and gay marriages have been controversial, making headline news. In 2004, Massachusetts became the first state to make same-sex marriages legal. In February 2004, the mayor of San Francisco issued marriage licenses to homosexual couples, which was halted by the California Supreme Court in March 2004.

- *ROE V. WADE.* In 1973 the Supreme Court's landmark decision to legally allow women to have an abortion gave women a newfound freedom of choice. This famous case began in Texas, when a pregnant woman, referred to as Jane Roe, filed suit against District Attorney Henry Wade. The state was preventing Roe from having an abortion and she was challenging the decision. Roe won and Wade appealed to the Supreme Court, which upheld the decision.

- ACCESS TO THE INTERNET. The Internet has exposed us to unlimited information about sex. Whether it's an atypical fetish or the answers to a set of sexual symptoms you are experiencing, the Internet is a ready source of information and has been a key factor in women's ability to advocate for their general and sexual health needs. There are chat rooms, medical Q and A's, and support groups all relating to sexuality.

- PUBLIC AWARENESS OF CHILDHOOD SEXUAL ABUSE. In the past, women who were victims of abuse were afraid to come forward for fear they wouldn't be believed. But by the 1970s attitudes began to change. With greater awareness of childhood physical abuse, childhood sexual abuse started to gain greater public consciousness. Therapists became much more aware of the signs of childhood sexual abuse and victims began recalling repressed memories in treatment. Support groups and social series addressing this issue started popping up. This allowed women to come forward and openly talk about the sexual trauma they experienced in childhood, allowing for further empowerment of women. In 1974 the Child Abuse Prevention and Treatment Act was signed. In 1977 the National Center of Child Abuse and Neglect developed child protection user manuals to guide professionals.

More recent was the scandal involving priests and young parishioners. Children who were abused by clergy were coming forward, demanding that their perpetrators be held accountable for their acts of sexual abuse.

- **SEX EDUCATION IN THE SCHOOLS.** Back in the 1950s, when sex education was taught in hygiene class, boys and girls were separated. The education consisted largely of what to expect in puberty, the anatomy of the male and female body, and reproduction. We have come a long way. Today's discussion often includes using protection, condom usage, and in some schools, although controversial, the passing out of condoms. The condom distribution was a result of the AIDS crisis and a campaign for safer sex.

- **ADVENT OF THE BIRTH CONTROL PILL.** In 1960 the Food and Drug Administration approved "the pill." This little tablet became the foundation of the sexual revolution. It became a radical new way to avoid pregnancy. A woman who popped the pill once a day could engage in sex without the fear of pregnancy.

- **WOMEN'S LIBERATION MOVEMENT.** The 1960s was a big turning point for women. Prior to that, American attitudes were that a woman's place should be in the home. Women were made to feel guilty if they didn't stay home to take care of their children, and those who did go to work were discriminated against and received lower pay. Women were fed up with being second-class citizens and being treated like sex objects. They were tired of being denied the same rights as men and wanted to change their status in society. They wanted to raise consciousness. And they did. The Women's Movement became one of the biggest social movements in the history of the country. While the struggle for women's rights was hardly new—the Women's Suffrage Movement started at the end of the nineteenth century—things had quieted down. Women burned their bras and feminism, sexism, and male chauvinism entered into mainstream vocabulary.

In 1966 the National Organization for Women (NOW) was formed. Their goal was to seek equality for men and women, especially in public life, labor laws, and employment.

- SEXUAL POLITICS. It's been said that many U.S. presidents have been unfaithful to their wives. However, presidential staffers have tried to keep the indiscretions under wraps. That all changed when Bill Clinton's sexual encounters with Monica Lewinsky became headline news worldwide. It also had people talking about the definition of sex. Was oral sex still sex? It brought the semantics of sex into question and raised a whole new consciousness.

  A sign of the times, despite his indiscretions, Clinton remained a popular president. Although his morals were under scrutiny, public opinion still showed that the American people, by and large, were forgiving. That was a far cry from not many years back when then–presidential hopeful Gary Hart was found cheating on his wife on the infamous boat *Monkey Business*. That cost him the nomination. The tide shifted in this country, becoming more accepting, or perhaps more immune, to infidelity and various types of sexual behavior.

- PLANNED PARENTHOOD. In 1916 Margaret Sanger, her sister, Ethel Byrne, and Fania Mindell opened the first birth control clinic in America, offering contraceptive information. It was housed in Brooklyn, New York. In 1942 the Birth Control Federation of America voted to change the name to Planned Parenthood. Since then it has continued to be a front-runner for the advocacy of women and the prevention of pregnancy and STDs. In recent years it has counseled young women on safe sex and tested them for AIDS. The right-to-lifers have protested Planned Parenthood for their pro-abortion stand.

- SEX IN THE MEDIA AND MUSIC. Back in the 1950s, when *I Love Lucy* was on the air, Lucy and Ricky couldn't be shown sleeping in the same bed. They couldn't even mention the word *pregnancy* when she was about to give birth on the show and in real life. Today, television viewers can choose from hundreds of stations on cable, broadcasting everything from sitcoms spouting profanity to explicit sex on select channels. Even on the big three networks, ABC's, NBC's, and CBS's steamy soap operas on daytime TV leave little to the imagination. The very popular sitcom *Seinfeld* had an episode all about masturbation. HBO's *Sex and the City* had millions of Americans running home on Sunday nights to see the sexual exploits of the four New York City–dwelling thirty-something beauties. What was once considered unspeakable became a story line on TV.

Music, too, has made its impression on the younger generation. Britney Spears's and Madonna's scanty attire is quite a leap from Rosemary Clooney's in the 1950s. Today's lyrics, especially rap music, are no holds barred.

Final Thoughts

We set out to find the characteristics of a sexually satisfied woman, and learned that any one of us can be sexually satisfied. We learned that age wasn't a factor, and neither was race, ethnicity, religion, or having children. We were pleased to discover that the percentage of sexually satisfied women was higher than we anticipated. And the good news is that it's a large number—74.4 percent of women in America report that they are sexually satisfied. It's also promising that it made no difference if you were rich or poor, married or single, have one sexual partner or twenty. It doesn't matter if you have more conservative attitudes about sex or less conservative ones. And believe it or not, while it's nice when it happens, orgasm is not the key to women's sexual satisfaction!

What can we learn from these sexually satisfied women? What do they have in common? Well, first of all they feel their sex lives work, in terms of function and response. They are confident and know how to advocate for their sexual needs. They believe men and women both deserve sexual pleasure. They feel happy and contented in a life they experience as exciting, and they feel good about the way they look. They believe in their sexual abilities in the bedroom and communicate their sexual desires and needs to their partners. They enjoy masturbation and do so alone as well as with their partners.

What's similar about the partners and relationships of these lucky women? First and foremost, size does seem to matter. Sexually satisfied women report that their partners' penises are on the larger side. It seems that age-old myth isn't a myth after all. Sexually satisfied women also enjoy active social lives and feel close to their partners and share a sense of emotional intimacy with them. As important as physical response may be, over 80 percent of all the women surveyed, satisfied or not, feel that sex should not happen without love. In our first book, *For Women Only,* we talked about the inherent differences between men and women and how they experience sex. All of our clinical work and research over the years has highlighted the importance of the context in which a woman experiences her sexuality. The findings of the Women's Sexual Satisfaction Survey support what we have always known: Sexual response and enjoyment are crucial, but how we feel about ourselves, our bodies, and the person we are with are the keys to our ability to feel satisfied.

We have tried to provide some key clues into how to optimize your sex life and reach sexual satisfaction. We truly believe that there is a sexually satisfied woman in every one of us. We just have to be willing to do the work and take the risks that are involved in letting her out. The key may be simple, or more complex. You may have to challenge belief systems you've carried with you throughout your life, turn your relationship upside down, or take emotional risks that require a great deal of courage. But we believe the journey is well worth it. Hopefully this book will give you some stepping-stones to get started. We wish you luck and a pleasant and productive journey!

Appendix

Notes

Chapter 1: Communication In and Out of the Bedroom

Maltz, Wendy. *In the Garden of Desire* (New York: Broadway Books, 1998).

Chapter 2: Emotional Well-being

Branden, Nathaniel. *The Six Pillars of Self-Esteem* (New York: Bantam Doubleday Dell, 1994).

Cohen, Sheldon, Ph.D. "Reactivity and Vulnerability to Stress-Associated Risk for Upper Respiratory Illness." *Psychosomatic Medicine* 64 (2002): 302–310. Published by the American Psychosomatic Society.

Davis, Michele Weiner. *The Sex-Starved Marriage: A Couple's Guide to Boosting Their Marriage Libido* (New York: Simon & Schuster, 2003), p. 80.

Fisher, Helen. *The First Sex* (New York: Ballantine, 2000).

Folkers, Gladys, and Jeanne Engelmann. *Taking Charge of My Mind and Body: A Girl's Guide to Outsmarting Alcohol, Drugs, Smoking, and Eating Problems* (Minneapolis, Minn.: Free Spirit Publishing, 1997).

Geracioti Jr., Thomas D., M.D. "Persistent Depression? Low Libido? Think Testosterone Deficiency." *Current Psychiatry* (May 2004): 26.

Jones, Jeffrey M. "Little Change in Americans' Stress Levels Over Last Eight Years." *Gallup Poll Monthly,* no. 436 (January 2002): 43–45.

Minchinton, Jerry. *Maximum Self-Esteem: The Handbook for Reclaiming Your Sense of Self-Worth* (Van Zant, Miss.: Arnford House Publishers, 1993), p. 27.

Phillips Jr., Robert, M.D., and James R. Slaughter, M.D. "Depression and Sexual Desire," *American Family Physician* (August 15, 2000). Published by the American Academy of Family Physicians.

Redmond, Laure. *Feel Good Naked* (Gloucester, Mass.: Fair Winds Press, 2002), p. 23.

Wiederman, Michael. "Women's Body Image Self-Consciousness During Physical Intimacy with a Partner." *The Journal of Sex Research* 37 (February 2000): 60.

Chapter 3: Relationship Health

Behrendt, Greg, and Liz Tuccillo. *He's Just Not That Into You* (New York: Simon & Schuster, 2004), pp. 23, 79.

Cain, Virginia. "Sexual Functioning and Practices," *Journal of Sex Research* 40, no. 3 (August 2003): 266–276. Swan Study, National Institutes of Health Study of Women's Health Across the Nation.

Clement, Christy, and Kay McLean. *Wired Not Weird: A Woman's Guide to Dating Online* (Synergetic Publications, 2000), pp. 38, 60, 65.

Fisher, Helen E. *Anatomy of Love* (New York: Fawcett Books, 1992), pp. 57, 162.

———. *The Sex Contract: The Evolution of Human Behavior* (New York: William Morrow, 1983).

———. *Why We Love: The Nature and Chemistry of Romantic Love* (New York: Henry Holt, 2004).

Schnarch, David, Ph.D. *Passionate Marriage: Keeping Love and Intimacy Alive in Committed Relationships* (New York: Henry Holt, 1997), p. 160.

Shelburne, Walter A., Ph.D. *For Play: 150 Sex Games for Couples* (Oakland, Calif.: Waterfall Press, 1993), pp. 27, 32, 37, 40, 59, 127.

Chapter 4: Self-stimulation

Chalker, Rebecca. *The Clitoral Truth* (New York: Seven Stories Press, 2000), p. 150.

Dodson, Betty. *Orgasms for Two* (New York: Crown Publishing, 2002).

Maltz, Wendy. *In the Garden of Desire* (New York: Broadway Books, 1998).

Rosenau, Dr. Douglas E. *A Celebration of Sex* (Nashville, Tenn.: Thomas Nelson Publishers, 2002), p. 224.

Chapter 5: Arousal, Lubrication, and Orgasm

Berman, Jennifer, M.D., and Laura Berman, Ph.D. *For Women Only: A Revolutionary Guide to Reclaiming Your Sex Life* (New York: Henry Holt, 2001), pp. 48, 158.

Davis, Michele Weiner. *The Sex-Starved Marriage: A Couple's Guide to Boosting Their Marriage Libido* (New York: Simon & Schuster, 2003), p. 38.

Schnarch, David, Ph.D. *Passionate Marriage: Keeping Love and Intimacy Alive in Committed Relationships* (New York: Henry Holt, 1997).

Weeks, Gerald R., and Nancy Gambescia. *Hypoactive Sexual Desire* (New York: W.W. Norton & Company, 2002).

Chapter 6: Addressing Your Past

Bart, Pauline B., and Eileen Geil Moran. *In Violence Against Women: The Bloody Footprints* (Thousand Oaks, Calif.: Sage Publications, 1993), p. 48.

Bass, Ellen, and Laura Davis. *The Courage to Heal: A Guide for Women Survivors of Child Sexual Abuse* (New York: HarperPerennial, 1994).

Berman, Jennifer, M.D., and Laura Berman, Ph.D. *For Women Only: A Revolutionary Guide to Reclaiming Your Sex Life* (New York: Henry Holt, 2001).

Patterson, C.H., and Suzanne C. Hidore. "The Primary Prevention of Psychosocial Disorders: A Person/Client Centered Perspective." *Person-Centered Journal* 4, no. 1 (1997).

Quigley, Ann. "Father's Absence Increases Daughter's Risk of Teen Pregnancy." *Health Behavior News Service,* May 14, 2003. Center for the Advancement of Health.

Weeks, Gerald R., and Nancy Gambescia. *Hypoactive Sexual Desire* (New York: W.W. Norton & Company, 2002).

White, Emily. *Fast Girls: Teenage Tribes and the Myth of the Slut* (New York: Scribner, 2002), p. 45.

Zolbrod, Aline P., Ph.D. *Sex Smart: How Your Childhood Shaped Your Sexual Life and What to Do About It* (Oakland, Calif.: New Harbinger Press, 1998), pp. 17, 119.

Chapter 7: Accepting and Overcoming Physical Obstacles

Arthritis Foundation. *A Guide to Intimacy with Arthritis* (Atlanta: Arthritis Foundation, 1998).

Charilfue, S.W. "Sexual Issues of Women with Spinal Cord Injuries," *Paraplegia* (March 30, 1992): 192–199.

Enzlin, Paul, Chantal Mathieu, Annick Van Den Bruel, et al. "Sexual Dysfunction in Women with Type 1 Diabetes: A Controlled Study." *Diabetes Care* (April 2002).

Kahn, Alice Lapas, Beverly Whipple, and John D. Perry. *The G Spot and Other Discoveries About Human Sexuality* (New York: Dell Publishing, 1983).

Karp, Gary. *Life on Wheels: For the Active Wheelchair User* (Sebastopol, Calif.: O'Reilly & Associates, Incorporated, 1998).

Laumann, E.O., A. Paik, and R.C. Rosen. "Sexual Dysfunction in the United States: Prevalence and Predictors." *Journal of the American Medical Association* 281 (1999): pp. 533–537.

Nausbaum, Margaret R.H., Carol Hamilton, and Patricia Lenahan. "Chronic Illness and Sexual Functioning." *American Family Physician* (January 15, 2003).

Schweiger, Alice Burdick. "Sleep Disorders." *Family Circle Magazine* (February 17, 2004): 108–111.

Slon, Stephanie. *Sexuality in Midlife and Beyond.* Edited by Alan Altman, M.D., and Suki Hanfling (Boston: Harvard Medical School, Harvard Health Publications, 2003).

Somers, Suzanne. *The Sexy Years* (New York: Crown Publishers, 2004), p. 45.

Peeters, Anna, Ph.D. "Obesity in Adulthood and Its Consequences for Life Expectancy: A Life-Table Analysis." *Annals of Internal Medicine* 138, no. 1 (January 2003): 24–32.

Chapter 8: Sexual Empowerment

Carnes, Patrick J. *Sexual Anorexia: Overcoming Sexual Self-Hatred* (Century City, Minn.: Hazelden Publishing & Educational Services, 1997).

Gunther, Bernard. *Sense Relaxation* (Franklin Lakes, N.J.: Career Press Incorporated, 1986).

Schnarch, David, Ph.D. *Passionate Marriage: Keeping Love and Intimacy Alive in Committed Relationships* (New York: Henry Holt, 1997), p. 86.

Chapter 9: Attitudes and Sex Across the Generations

Denizet-Lewis, Benoit. "Friends, Friends with Benefits and the Benefits of the Local Mall." *New York Times Magazine* (May 30, 2004): 32–34, 54.

Lunardini, Christine, Ph.D. *What Every American Should Know About Women's History: 200 Events That Shaped Our Destiny* (Holbrook, Mass.: Adams Media Corporation, 1997).

Michael, Robert T., John H. Gagnon, Edward O. Laumann, and Gina Kolata. *Sex in America: A Definitive Survey* (Boston: Little, Brown, 1994), p. 97.

Products

Lubricants

Many of our patients ask for suggestions for lubricants. These are some that we suggest:

Glycerin-based
Uberlube
Pjur
Women by Body Glide
Vitamin E
Vielle Lubricant

Water-based
Liquid Silk
Astroglide
KY jelly

You should be able to find the water-based lubricants listed at your local drugstore as well as some of the glycerin-based brands. Otherwise you can find them at erotica shops (see below).

Erotic Shopping and Sexual Information

These are some of the best-known female friendly resources for purchasing sexual aids and gathering sexual health information:

BETTY DODSON WORKSHOPS

For online advice, courses, videos, and books on self-stimulation and self-loving.
www.bettydodson.com

DRUGSTORE.COM

Offers a large selection of products on sexual aids on their sexual well-being page. Many people like having a package arrive that implies it's from a drugstore rather than an erotica shop.
www.drugstore.com

EVE'S GARDEN INTERNATIONAL

Online catalog offers a variety of sex toys, scented massage oils, erotic books and videos.
(800) 848-3837
www.eve'sgarden.com

GOOD VIBRATIONS

Online catalog specializing in vibrators, sex toys, and erotic books and videos.
(800) BUY-VIBE
www.goodvibes.com

GRAND OPENING! SEXUALITY BOUTIQUE

www.grandopening.com

MARRIAGE AND FAMILY HEALTH CENTER

Founded by Dr. David Schnarch and Dr. Ruth Morehouse, this center offers sexuality enhancement courses, retreats, and couples-enrichment weekends.
(303) 670-2630
www.passionatemarriage.com

MYPLEASURE

Complete selection of sex toys and advice on sex.
www.mypleasure.com

Suggested Reading

General/Couples Sexuality

Barbach, Lonnie, Ph.D. *For Each Other: Sharing Sexual Intimacy*. New York: Signet, 2001.

Chapman, Gary, and James S. Bell. *Five Love Languages: How to Express Heartfelt Commitment to Your Mate*. Chicago: Northfield Publishing, 1996.

Corn, Laura. *101 Nights of Grrreat Romance: How to Make Love with Your Clothes On*. Park Avenue Publishers, Inc., 1996.

Davis, Michele Weiner. *The Sex-Starved Marriage: A Couple's Guide to Boosting Their Marriage Libido*. New York: Simon & Schuster, 2003.

Dodson, Betty. *Orgasms for Two*. New York: Crown Publishing, 2002.

Fisher, Helen E. *Anatomy of Love: The Mysteries of Mating, Marriage, and Why We Stray*. New York: Fawcett Book Group, 1993.

Goddard, Jamie, and Kurt Brungardt. *Lesbian Sex Secrets for Men: What Every Man Wants to Know About Making Love to a Woman and Never Asks*. New York: Penguin Group, 2000.

Gottman, John, and Joan de Claire. *The Relationship Cure: A 5-Step Guide to Strengthening Your Marriage, Family, and Friendships*. New York: Random House, 2002.

Harley, Willard F. *His Needs, Her Needs: Building an Affair-Proof Marriage*. Grand Rapids, Mich.: Baker Book House, 2001.

Hendrix, Harville. *Keeping the Love You Find*. New York: Simon & Schuster, 1993.

Hutcherson, Hilda, M.D. *What Your Mother Never Told You About Sex*. New York: Berkeley Publishing Group, 2002.

Hutchinson, Marcia Germaine. *200 Ways to Love the Body You Have*. Freedom, Calif.: Crossing Press Inc., 1999.

Kaplan, H. S., and D. Passalacqua. *Illustrated Manual of Sex Therapy*. Philadelphia: Taylor & Francis, Inc. (paperback), 1988.

Love, Patricia, and Jo Robinson. *Hot Monogamy: Essential Steps to More Passionate, Intimate Lovemaking*. New York: Plume, 1995.

Paget, Lou. *The Big O: Orgasms: How to Have Them, Give Them, and Keep Them Coming*. New York: Broadway Books, 2001.

———. *How to Give Her Absolute Pleasure*. New York: Bantam Doubleday Dell, 2000.

———. *365 Days of Sensational Sex: Tantalizing Tips and Techniques for Keeping the Fires Burning All Year Long*. New York: Gotham, 2003.

———. *How to Be a Great Lover: Girlfriend-to-Girlfriend, Totally Explicit Techniques That Will Blow His Mind*. New York: Random House, 1999.

Rako, Susan. *The Hormone of Desire: The Truth About Testosterone, Sexuality, and Menopause*. New York: Crown Publishing, 1996.

Redmond, Laure. *Feel Good Naked: 10 No-Diet Secrets to a Fabulous Body*. Gloucester, Mass.: Fair Winds Press, 2002.

Schnarch, David. *Constructing the Sexual Crucible: An Integration of Sexual and Marital Therapy*. New York: W. W. Norton & Co., 1991.

———. *Passionate Marriage: Keeping Love and Intimacy Alive in Committed Relationships*. New York: Henry Holt, 1997.

Somers, Suzanne. *The Sexy Years*. New York: Crown Publishers, 2004.

Zolbrod, Aline P., Ph.D. *Sex Smart: How Your Childhood Shaped Your Sexual Life and What to Do About It*. New York: New Harbinger, 1998.

Female Sexuality

Barbach, Lonnie, Ph.D. *For Yourself: The Fulfillment of Female Sexuality*. New York: New American Library, 1991.

Berman, Jennifer, M.D., and Laura Berman, Ph.D. *For Women Only: A Revolutionary Guide to Reclaiming Your Sex Life*. New York: Henry Holt, 2001.

Chalker, Rebecca. *The Clitoral Truth: The Secret World at Your Fingertips*. New York: Seven Stories Press, 2000.

Dodson, Betty. *Sex for One: The Joy of Self Loving*. New York: Crown Publishing, 1996.

Goodwin, A. J., and M. E. Agronin. *A Woman's Guide to Overcoming Sexual Fear and Pain*. New York: New Harbinger, 1997.

Heiman, J., and J. Lo Piccolo. *Becoming Orgasmic: A Sexual and Personal Growth Program for Women*. New York: Simon & Schuster, 1988.

Male Sexuality

Kaplan, H. S. *How to Overcome Premature Ejaculation*. New York: Brunner Mazel, 1989.

Zilbergeld, B. *The New Male Sexuality: The Truth About Men, Sex and Pleasure*. New York: Bantam Doubleday Dell, 1999.

Sexual Abuse

Bass, Ellen, and Laura Davis. *The Courage to Heal: A Guide for Women Survivors of Child Sexual Abuse.* New York: HarperPerennial, 1994.

Davis, L. *Allies in Healing: When the Person You Love Was Sexually Abused as a Child, a Support Book.* New York: HarperPerennial, 1991.

Maltz, W. *The Sexual Healing Journey: A Guide for Survivors of Sexual Abuse.* New York: HarperPerennial, 1992.

Resources

Medical Organizations

AMERICAN CANCER SOCIETY

Provides an enormous amount of information, including cancer treatments, clinical trials, support groups, cancer facts and statistics, medical updates, and survivor stories.
www.cancer.org

AMERICAN DIABETES ASSOCIATION

Tips on such topics as living with diabetes, nutrition and recipes, diabetes research, and diabetes prevention.
www.diabetes.org

AMERICAN HEART ASSOCIATION

Offers a wealth of information about heart disease and stroke, including warning signs, statistics, who's at risk, healthy lifestyle tips, and dietary recommendations.
www.americanheart.org

ARTHRITIS FOUNDATION

Provides tips on living with arthritis, questions and answers, drug guide, facts and statistics, user-friendly products for arthritis sufferers, and more.
www.arthritis.org

SEXUAL HEALTH NETWORK

Provides resources for sexuality education, information, therapy, medical attentions for people with disabilities, illnesses, and health-related problems.
www.sexualhealth.com

VULVAR PAIN FOUNDATION

Provides information about vulvar pain and related disorders.
www.vulvarpainfoundation.org

Sexual Abuse

HEALING WOMAN FOUNDATION

This nonprofit organization provides recovery resources for women survivors of childhood sexual abuse.
(408) 246-1788
www.healingwoman.org

VOICES IN ACTION (VICTIMS OF INCEST CAN EMERGE SURVIVORS)

Provides assistance to adult victims of child abuse.
www.voices-action.org

General Health and Women's Issues

NATIONAL WOMEN'S HEALTH NETWORK

An advocacy group that works on different policies affecting women's health. Information clearinghouse—(202) 628-7814—provides packets and fact sheets on various women's health issues. They attend to specific health questions and research the answers.
www.nwhn.org

NORTH AMERICAN MENOPAUSE SOCIETY (NAMS)

This is a nonprofit organization helping women through and beyond menopause. It also provides information on perimenopause and estrogen loss.
(800) 774-5342 or (404) 442-7550
www.menopause.org

PLANNED PARENTHOOD

A long-established excellent resource for information about birth control, family planning, abortion, and women's health. They can help you find a clinic in your area.
(800) 230-PLAN
www.plannedparenthood.org

Therapy and Therapists

Finding an appropriate therapist isn't always an easy task. First and foremost in choosing a therapist, make sure he or she is a licensed mental health practitioner. Ask about education, training, certification, and specialty. For a referral, call your family physician, local hospital, nearby medical center or professional organization (listed below). Licensed therapists are typically clinical social workers, psychiatrists, psychologists, or marriage and family therapists. Here is what you should know:

- Clinical social workers have at least a master's degree (MSW) in social work and a minimum of two years of supervised experience. Some states require a license, some just registration. Professional organization: National Association of Social Workers (*www.naswdc.org*).
- Psychiatrists are medical doctors who have had four years of medical school and residency training in psychiatry. In most states they are the only mental health professionals able to prescribe medication. They need a state license to practice. Professional organization: American Psychiatric Association (*www.psych.org*).
- Psychologists can have either a Ph.D., an Ed.D., or a Psy.D., have served a one-year residency and a one-year clinical internship. They need a state license to practice independently. Professional organization: American Psychological Association (*www.apa.org*).
- Marriage and family therapists (MFTs) have at least a master's degree in marriage and family therapy and at least two years of supervised clinical training. Professional organization: American Association for Marriage and Family Therapy (*www.aamft.org*).

For types of therapy, consider individual psychotherapy, couples, or sex therapy:

- **General individual psychotherapy** addresses issues you have in your life and relationships that are based on emotional and/or historical factors. Dealing with a trauma history, coping with depression, anxiety, and difficulties in social or romantic relationships are often the focus of individual therapy. The work is typically focused on identifying negative patterns and messages and learning new, positive ways to cope and interact with others.
- **General couples therapy** focuses on problems in a relationship between two people. The goal is to help the couple identify conflicts, resolve the issues, and learn how to better communicate.
- **Sex therapy** is less clinical than general and couples therapy, and more educational, informative, and behavioral, typically involving homework. Sex therapy never involves having sex in the office—it is only talk therapy. Often sex therapy is incorporated into individual and couples therapy as a component of treatment. Sex therapists are psychologists, psychiatrists,

clinical social workers, or marriage and family therapists who specialize in problems and concerns relating to sexual function. They have had post-graduate training in sexual counseling. Sex therapy can be done as part of individual or couples work. If you are going to a sex therapist for couples issues, make sure he or she has had extensive experience and training in general couples therapy as well as sex therapy. Professional organization: The American Association of Sex Educators, Counselors and Therapists (AASECT.org.)

Websites

Internet Dating Websites

There are hundreds of websites designed to hook up singles looking for mates. According to the marketing research firm ComScore Media Metrix, these are some of the more popular ones:

Netscape love & personals
www.americansingles.com
www.cupidjunction.com
www.date.com
www.dreambook.com
www.eharmony.com
www.friendfinder.com
www.gay.com
www.great-expectations.net
www.imatchup.com
www.Jdate.com
www.lavalight.com
www.loveaccess.com
www.love.com
www.match.com
www.matchnet.com
www.one2match.com
www.relationshipexchange.com
www.seniorfriendfinder.com
www.someonelikesyou.com
Yahoo personals

Sexually Related Websites

American Association for Marriage and Family Therapy (AAMFT)
www.aamft.org

American Association of Sex Educators, Counselors, and Therapists (AASECT)
www.aasect.org

American Psychological Association (APA)
www.apa.org

American Psychological Society (APS)
www.hanover.edu/psych/APS/aps.html

His and Her Health
www.hisandherhealth.com

Kinsey Institute for Research in Sex, Gender and Reproduction
www.indiana.edu/~kinsey/

National Council on Family Relations (NCFR)
www.ncfr.com/body.html

Network for Excellence in Women's Sexual Health (NEWSHE)
www.newshe.com

Sexuality Information and Education Council of the United States (SIECUS)
www.siecus.org

The Society for the Scientific Study of Sexuality (SSSS)
www.ssc.wisc.edu/sss/

World Association for Sexology (WAS)
www.tc.umn.edu/nlhome/m201/colem001/was/

The Women's Sexual Satisfaction Survey

Description of Survey Methods

The telephone survey data were collected by REDA International, located in Wheaton, Maryland, between April 30 and July 31, 2003, from a national sample of 2,604 American women between the ages of eighteen and seventy-one. REDA used a random digit dial sampling procedure to select numbers and attempted to call these numbers between the hours of ten A.M. and nine P.M., Monday through Saturday. They made up to 18 attempts to reach each sampled number with an average of 3.7 attempts per number. Calculated according to the formula specified by the Council of American Survey Research Organizations, the response rate for the survey was 13 percent, calculated using the formula: response rate = number of completes / (known eligibles + presumed eligibles among the numbers where true eligibility could not be established). Calls were made from the REDA central computerized telephone interviewing center. Interviewers for this study were females and each received six hours of training prior to interviewing.

Post-stratification weights were formed on the basis of race-ethnicity (Hispanic, non-Hispanic white, African-American/Other), education (less than high school, high school grad/GED, some college/2-year degree, 4-year degree, master's degree and above), and age (18–24/25–34/35–44/45–54/55–64/65–71), using the 2000 U.S. Census totals. The resultant weights, which mainly corrected for under-representation of Hispanics, those with "Other" ethnicities, those under 45, and those with less than a high school education, resulted in a moderate design effect of 1.28, which was accounted for in all analyses.

The interview content was developed with consultation from staff of The RAND Corporation in Santa Monica, California. Sources of items used in the survey include the interview used for the National Health and Social Life survey and sexual satisfaction scales adapted from scales developed by Derogatis and Melisaratos (1979) and Young and Luquis (1998) and the RAND measures of general health and mental health available on the RAND website at http://www.rand.org/health/surveys.html.

Derogatis, L. R., and N. Melisaratos. "The DSFI: A Multidimensional Measure of Sexual Functioning." *Journal of Sex and Marital Therapy* 5 (1979):244–281.

Lauman, Edward O., John H. Gagnon, Robert T. Michael, and Stuart Michaels. *The Social Organization of Sexuality: Sexual Practices in the United States.* Chicago: University of Chicago Press, 1994.

Young, Michael, and Raffy Luquis. "Correlates of Sexual Satisfaction in Marriage." *Canadian Journal of Human Sexuality* 7, no. 2 (1998):115–27.

The Questionnaire

Section A: Sexual Attitudes

First, we'd like to ask you some questions about your attitudes toward sex.

A1. In general, how important is having a satisfying sex life to you? Would you say it is?

    4   Very important
    3   Somewhat important
    2   A little bit important, OR
    1   Not important at all
    5   (DK—Don't Know)
    6   (Refused)

A2. There's been a lot of discussion about the way morals and attitudes about sex are changing in this country. If a man and a woman have sex relations before marriage, do you think it is?

    4   Always wrong
    3   Almost always wrong
    2   Wrong only sometimes
    1   Not wrong at all
    5   (DK)
    6   (Refused)

A3. What if they are in their teens, say 14 to 16 years old? In that case, do you think sex relations before marriage are?

    4   Always wrong
    3   Almost always wrong
    2   Wrong only sometimes
    1   Not wrong at all
    5   (DK)
    6   (Refused)

A4. What is your opinion about a married person having sexual relations with someone other than the marriage partner. Is it?

    4   Always wrong
    3   Almost always wrong
    2   Wrong only sometimes
    1   Not wrong at all
    5   (DK)
    6   (Refused)

A5. What is your opinion about sexual relations between two adults of the same sex? Do you think it is?

    4   Always wrong
    3   Almost always wrong
    2   Wrong only sometimes
    1   Not wrong at all
    5   (DK)
    6   (Refused)

A6. I would not have sex with someone unless I was in love with him or her.

    4   Strongly agree
    3   Agree
    2   Disagree
    1   Strongly disagree

F. C
G. D
H. A

F10. Have
lowing?
1   Y
2   N
3   (I
4   (F
A. H
    oc
B. Ba
C. Ve
    a
D. In
E. Su
    ut

F11. Are y
kinds of m
ing drugs
blood pres
urinary inc
1   Yes
2   No
3   (D
4   (R

Section
Finally, we
questions
sponses.

G1. What y
9998 (D
9999 (R

5   (DK)
6   (Refused)

A7. My religious beliefs have shaped and guided my sexual behavior.
4   Strongly agree
3   Agree
2   Disagree
1   Strongly disagree
5   (DK)
6   (Refused)

Section B: Sexual Health History

B1. In general, over the past 12 months, would you say your sex life has been:
6   Excellent
5   Very good
4   Good
3   Fair
2   Poor
1   Very poor
7   (Didn't have any sex life past 12 months)
8   (DK)
9   (Refused)

B2. Have you ever *in your life* had an orgasm from any kind of sex, including sex with another person or from you touching yourself?
1   Yes
2   No
3   (Not sure)
4   (DK)
5   (Refused)

People mean different things by sex or sexual activity, but in answering the next several questions we need every-

one to use the same definition. Here, by "sex" we mean any activity with another person that was okay with both of you and involved touching genitals and feeling sexually excited, even if intercourse or orgasm did not happen.

B3. Have you ever had sex with another person, including sex that turned you on even if there was no actual intercourse or orgasm?
1   Yes
2   No
3   (Not sure)
4   (DK)
5   (Refused)

B4. People have many reasons for not being sexually active, please tell me the main reasons you have never been sexually active.
1   Other (list)
2   (DK)
3   (Refused)
4   Never had a partner
5   Religious reasons
6   Not interested
7   Physical problem

B5. Have you ever had vaginal intercourse, that is, a man put his penis into your vagina, when you wanted him to do that?
1   Yes
2   No
3   (Not sure)
4   (DK)
5   (Refused)

G5. Last year, in 2002, was your total family income from all sources over or under $20,000?

> Was it over or under $10,000?
> Was it over or under $35,000?
> Was it over or under $50,000?
> Was it over or under $75,000?
> 1 Less than $10,000
> 2 $10,000 to less than $20,000
> 3 $20,000 to less than $35,000
> 4 $35,000 to less than $50,000
> 5 $50,000 to less than $75,000
> 6 $75,000 or more

G6. We are interested in how people are getting along financially these days. So far as you (and your family) are concerned, would you say you are pretty well satisfied with your present financial situation, more or less satisfied, or not satisfied at all?

> 3 Pretty well satisfied
> 2 More or less satisfied
> 1 Not satisfied at all
> 4 (DK)
> 5 (Refused)

G7. How important would you say religion or spirituality is to your life?

> 4 Very important
> 3 Somewhat important
> 2 A little bit important
> 1 Not important at all

> 5 (DK)
> 6 (Refused)

G8. How many children have you ever had? Please count all that were born alive at any time, including any from previous marriages or relationships.

> 98 (DK)
> 99 (Refused)

G9. Do you currently have children age 18 or under living in your household, including your own children or any other children?

> 1 Yes
> 2 No
> 3 (DK)
> 4 (Refused)

G10. Have you ever been married or lived with someone in a sexual relationship for a month or more?

> 1 Yes
> 2 No
> 3 (DK)
> 4 (Refused)

G11. Are you now married or are you living with someone in a sexual relationship that has lasted for a month or more?

> 1 Yes
> 2 No
> 3 (DK)
> 4 Refused

PADDINGTON
HERE AND NOW

Other Paddington Storybooks by Michael Bond

A Bear Called Paddington
More About Paddington
Paddington Abroad
Paddington Helps Out
Paddington at Large
Paddington Marches On
Paddington at Work
Paddington Takes the Air
Paddington on Top
Paddington Takes the Test
Paddington on Screen

PADDINGTON
HERE AND NOW

by MICHAEL BOND

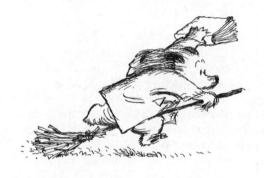

illustrated by R.W. Alley

HarperCollins*Publishers*

Library of Congress Cataloging-in-Publication Data is available.
ISBN 978-0-06-147364-7 (trade bdg.)
ISBN 978-0-06-147365-4 (lib. bdg.)

1 2 3 4 5 6 7 8 9 10
❖
First U.S. edition, HarperCollins Publishers Inc., 2008
First published in Great Britain by HarperCollins Publishers Ltd.
in 2008

CONTENTS

1. PARKING PROBLEMS   1

2. PADDINGTON'S GOOD TURN   23

3. PADDINGTON STRIKES A CHORD   46

4. PADDINGTON TAKES THE CAKE   71

5. PADDINGTON SPILLS THE BEANS   95

6. PADDINGTON AIMS HIGH   119

7. PADDINGTON'S CHRISTMAS SURPRISE   141

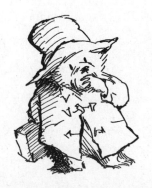

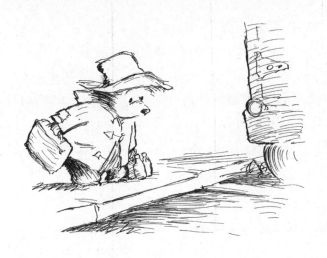

Chapter One

PARKING PROBLEMS

"MY SHOPPING BASKET on wheels has been towed away!" exclaimed Paddington hotly.

He gazed at the spot where he had left it before going into the cut-price grocer's in the Portobello Market. In all the years he had lived in London such a thing had never happened to him before, and he could hardly believe his eyes. But if he thought staring at the empty space was going to make it reappear, he was doomed to disappointment.

"It's coming to something if a young bear gent can't leave 'is shopping basket unattended for five minutes while 'e's going about 'is business," said one of the stall holders who normally supplied Paddington with vegetables when he was out shopping for the Brown family. "I don't know what the world's coming to."

"There's no give and take anymore," agreed a man at the next stall. "It's all take and no give. They'll be towing *us* away next, you mark my words."

"You should have left a note on it saying 'Back in five minutes,'" said a third one.

"Fat lot of good that would have done," said another. "They don't give you five seconds these days, let alone five minutes."

Paddington was a popular figure in the market, and by now a small crowd of sympathizers had begun to gather. Although he was known to drive a hard bargain, he was much respected by the traders. Receiving his business was regarded by many as being something of an honor—on a par with having a sign saying they were by appointment to a member of the royal family.

"The foreman of the truck said it was in the way of his vehicle," said a lady who had witnessed the event. "They were trying to get behind a car they wanted to tow away."

"But my buns were in it," said Paddington.

"'*Were*' is probably the right word," replied the lady. "I daresay even now they're parked in some side street or other wolfing them down. Driving those great big tow-away trucks of theirs must give them an appetite."

"I don't know what Mr. Gruber is going to say when he hears," said Paddington. "They were meant for our elevenses."

"Look on the bright side," said another lady. "At least you've still got your suitcase with you. The basket could have been clamped. That would have cost you eighty pounds to get it undone."

"And you would have to hang about half the day before they got around to doing it," agreed another.

Paddington's face grew longer and longer as he listened to all the words of wisdom. "Eighty pounds!" he exclaimed. "But I only went in for Mrs. Bird's bottled water!"

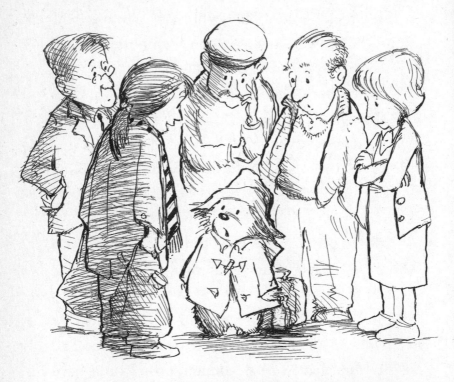

"You can buy a new basket on wheels in the market for ten pounds," chimed in another stall holder.

"I daresay if you haggle a bit you could get one for a lot less," said another.

"But I've only got ten pence," said Paddington sadly. "Besides, I wouldn't want a new one. Mr. Brown gave mine to me soon after I arrived. I've had it ever since."

"Quite right!" agreed an onlooker. "You stick to your guns. They don't come like that these days. Them new ones is all plastic. Don't last five minutes."

"If you ask me," said a lady who ran a knickknacks stall, "it's a pity it *didn't* get clamped. My Sid would have lent you his hacksaw like a shot. He doesn't hold with that kind of thing."

"Pity you weren't here in person when they did it," said another stall holder. "You would have been able to lie down in the road in front of their truck as a protest. Then we could have phoned the local press to send over one of their photographers, and it would have been in all the papers."

"That would have stopped the lorry in its tracks," agreed someone else from the back of the crowd.

Paddington eyed the man doubtfully. "Supposing it didn't?" he said.

"In that case you would have been on the

evening news," said the man. "Television would have had a field day interviewing all the witnesses."

"You'd have become what they call a martyr," agreed the first man. "I daresay in years to come they would have erected a statue in your honor. Then nobody would have been able to park."

"What you need," said the fruit-and-vegetable man, summing up the whole situation, "is a good lawyer. Someone like Sir Bernard Crumble. He lives just up the road. This kind of thing is just up his street. He's a great one for sticking up for the underdog—" He broke off as he caught Paddington's eye. "Well, I daresay he does under*bears* as well. He'd have their guts for garters. Never been known to lose a case yet."

"Which street does he live in?" asked Paddington hopefully.

"I shouldn't get ideas above your station," warned another trader, "if you'll pardon the pun. They do say 'e charges an arm and a leg just to open 'is front door to the postman."

"If I were you," said a passerby, "before you do anything else, I suggest you go along to the police station and report the matter to them. I daresay they'll be able to arrange counseling for you."

"Whatever you do," advised one of the stall holders, "don't tell them you've been towed away. Be what they call noncommittal. Just say your vehicle has gone missing."

He gazed at the large pack of bottled water Paddington had bought at the grocer's. "You can leave those with me. I'll make sure they don't come to any harm."

Paddington thanked the man for his kind offer and, after waving good-bye to the crowd, set off at a brisk pace toward the nearest police station.

But as he turned a corner and a familiar blue lamp came into view, he began to slow down. Over the years he had met a number of policemen, and he had always found them only too ready to help in times of trouble. There was the occasion when he'd mistaken a television repairman for a burglar, and another time when he had bought some oil shares from a man in the market and they had turned out to be duds.

But he had never actually gone into a police station all by himself before; and not knowing what to expect, he began to wish he had consulted his friend Mr. Gruber before taking the plunge. Mr. Gruber was always ready to help, and he most certainly would have done so had he heard their buns were missing. He might even have closed his shop for the morning.

And if he couldn't do that for any reason, there was always Mrs. Bird. Mrs. Bird looked after the Browns, and she didn't stand for any nonsense, especially if she thought Paddington was being hard done by.

However, as things turned out, he was pleasantly surprised when he mounted the steps and pushed the door slightly ajar. Apart from a man in uniform behind a counter, the room was completely empty.

The man was much younger than he had expected. In fact, he didn't seem much older than Mr. and Mrs. Brown's son, Jonathan, who was still at school. He looked slightly apprehensive when he caught sight of Paddington, rather as though he didn't know quite what to make of him.

"Er . . . *Sprechen Sie Deutsch?*" he ventured nervously.

"Bless you," said Paddington, politely raising his hat. "You can borrow my handkerchief if you like."

The policeman gave him a funny look before trying again.

"*Parlez-vous Français?*"

"Not today, thank you," said Paddington.

"Pardon me for asking," said the officer. "But it's Be Polite to Foreigners Week. Strictly unofficial, of course. It's the sergeant's idea, because we get a lot of overseas visitors at this time of the year, especially around the Portobello Road area, and I thought perhaps . . ."

"I'm not a foreigner," exclaimed Paddington hotly. "I'm from Darkest Peru."

The policeman looked put out. "Well, if that doesn't make you a foreigner, I don't know what does," he said. "Mind you, it takes all sorts. I must say, you speak very good English, wherever you're from."

"My Aunt Lucy taught me before she went into the Home for Retired Bears in Lima," said Paddington.

"Well, she did a good job, I'll say that for her," said the policeman. "What can we do for you?"

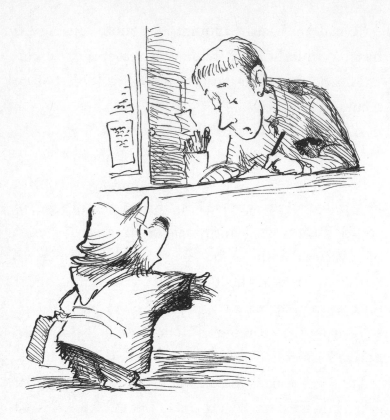

"I've come to see you about my vehicle," said
Paddington, choosing his words with care. "It isn't
where I left it."

"And where was that?" asked the policeman.

"Outside the cut-price grocer's in the market,"
said Paddington. "I always leave it there when I'm
out shopping."

"Oh, dear," said the officer. "Not another one gone missing. There's a lot of it about at the moment, especially around these parts." He reached for a computer keyboard. "I'd better take down some details."

"It had my buns in it," said Paddington.

"That's not a lot to go on," said the policeman. "I was wondering what make it is?"

"It's not really a make," said Paddington vaguely. "Mr. Brown built it for me when I first went to stay with them."

"Homemade," said the officer, typing in the words. "Ahhhhh! Color?"

"I think it's called wickerwork," said Paddington.

"I'll put down yellow for the time being," said the man. "Did you leave the hand brake on? That always slows them down a bit when they want to make a quick getaway."

"It doesn't have a hand brake," said Paddington. "It doesn't even have a paw brake. If I need to stop on a hill, I usually put some stones under the wheels. Especially if I've been to get the potatoes."

"Potatoes?" echoed the policeman. "What have

potatoes got to do with it?"

"They weigh a lot," explained Paddington. "Especially King Edwards. If my vehicle started to roll down a hill, I don't know what I would do. I expect I would close my eyes in case it hit something and all the potatoes fell out."

The policeman looked up from his keyboard and stared at Paddington. "I'll pretend I didn't hear that," he said, not unkindly. "That sort of thing wouldn't go down too well if it was read out in court. You might find yourself ending up in prison."

"Mind you," he continued. "It's probably on its way to Czechoslovakia or somewhere like that by now."

"Czechoslovakia!" exclaimed Paddington hotly. "But it's only just gone ten o'clock."

"You'd be surprised," said the man. "These people don't lose any time. A quick going over with a spray gun. Who knows what color it is by now. A new number plate . . . On the other hand, we don't let the grass grow under our feet." He picked up a telephone. "I'll put out an all-stations call."

"I don't have one of those," said Paddington, looking most relieved.

"One of what?" asked the policeman, holding his hand over the mouthpiece.

"A number plate," said Paddington.

The policeman replaced the receiver. "Hold on a minute," he said. "You'll be telling me next you haven't renewed your road tax."

"I haven't," said Paddington. He stared back at the man with growing excitement. It really was uncanny the way he knew about all the things he hadn't got.

"I'm glad I came here," he said. "I didn't know you had to pay taxes."

"Ignorance of the law is no excuse," said the policeman sternly. Reaching under the counter, he produced a large card showing a selection of pictures.

"I take it you are conversant with road signs."

Paddington peered at the card. "We didn't have anything like that in Darkest Peru," he said. "But there's one near where I live."

The policeman pointed at random to one of the

pictures. "What does that one show?"

"A man trying to open an umbrella," said Paddington promptly. "I expect it means it's about to rain."

"It's meant to depict a man with a shovel," said the policeman wearily. "That means there are road works ahead. If you ask me, you need to read your Highway Code again. Unless, of course—"

"You're quite right," broke in Paddington, more than ever pleased he had come to the police station. "I've never read it."

"I think it's high time I saw your driving license," said the policeman.

"I haven't got one of those either," exclaimed Paddington excitedly.

"Insurance?"

"What's that?" asked Paddington.

"What's that?" repeated the policeman. "*What's that?*"

He ran his fingers around the inside of his collar. The room had suddenly become very hot. "You'll be telling me next," he said, "that you haven't even passed your driving test."

"You're quite right," said Paddington excitedly. "I took it once by mistake, but I didn't pass because I drove into the examiner's car. I was in Mr. Brown's car at the time, and I had it in reverse by mistake. I don't think he was very pleased."

"Examiners are funny that way," said the policeman. "Bears like you are a menace to other road users."

"Oh, I never go on the road," said Paddington. "Not unless I have to. I always stick to the sidewalk."

The policeman gave him a long, hard look. He seemed to have grown older in the short time Paddington had been there. "You do realize," he said, "that I could throw the book at you."

"I hope you don't," said Paddington earnestly. "I'm not very good at catching things. It isn't easy with paws."

The policeman looked nervously over his shoulder before reaching into his back pocket.

"Talking of paws," he said casually, as he came around to the front of the counter. "Would you mind holding yours out in front of you?"

Paddington did as he was bid, and to his surprise

there was a click and he suddenly found his wrists held together by some kind of chain.

"I hope you have a good lawyer," said the policeman. "You're going to need one. You won't have a leg to stand on otherwise."

"I shan't have a leg to stand on?" repeated Paddington in alarm. He gave the man a hard stare. "But I had two when I came in!"

"I'm going to take your dabs now," said the policeman.

"My *dabs*!" repeated Paddington in alarm.

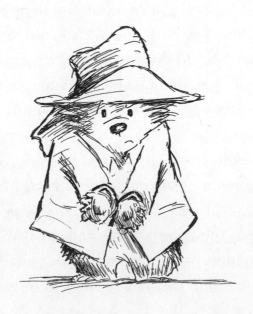

"Fingerprints," explained the policeman. "Only in your case I suppose we shall have to make do with paws. First of all I want you to press one of them down on this ink pad, then on some paper, so that we have a record of it for future reference."

"Mrs. Bird won't be very pleased if it comes off on the sheets," said Paddington.

"After that," said the policeman, ignoring the interruption, "you are allowed one telephone call."

"In that case," said Paddington, "I would like to ring Sir Bernard Crumble. He lives near here. He's supposed to very good on motoring offenses. I don't know if he does shopping baskets on wheels, but if he does, they told me in the market that he will have your guts for garters."

The policeman stared at him. "Did I hear you say shopping basket on wheels?' he exclaimed. "Why ever didn't you tell me that in the first place?"

"You didn't ask me," said Paddington. "I have a special license for it. It was given to me when I failed my driving test in a car. They said it would last me all my life. I expect Sir Bernard will want to see it. I keep it in a secret compartment of my suitcase. I can show it to you if you like. At least I could if I had it with me and I was able to use my paws."

He stared at the policeman, who seemed to have gone a pale shade of white. "Is anything the matter?" he asked. "Would you like a marmalade sandwich? I keep one under my hat in case of an emergency."

The policeman shook his head. "No, thank you." He groaned as he removed the handcuffs. "It's my first week on duty. They told me I might have some difficult customers to deal with, but I didn't think it would start quite so soon."

"I can come back later if you like," said Paddington hopefully.

"I'd much rather you didn't—" began the policeman. He broke off as a door opened and an older man came into the room. He had some stripes on his sleeve, and he looked very important.

"Ah," said the man, consulting a piece of paper he was holding. "Bush hat . . . blue duffle coat . . . Wellington boots . . . fits the description I was given over the phone . . . you must be the young gentleman who's had trouble with his shopping basket on wheels."

He turned to the first policeman. "You did well to keep him talking, Finsbury. Full marks."

"It was nothing, Sarge," said the constable, who seemed to have got some of his color back.

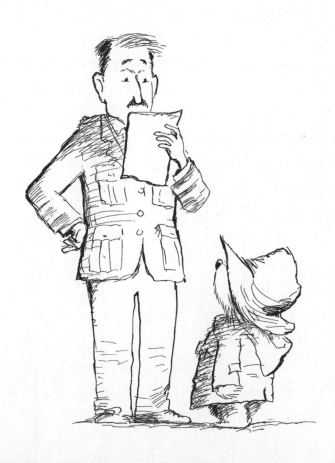

"It seems there's been a bit of a mix-up with the lads in the tow-away department," continued the sergeant, turning back to Paddington. "They put your basket on their vehicle for safekeeping while they were removing a car and forgot to take it off again. It went back to the depot with them.

"They've put some fresh buns in it for you. Apparently, somehow or other the ones that were in it got lost *en route*. Even now the basket's on its way back to where you left it. And there's nothing to pay. What do you say to that?"

"Thank you very much, Mr. Sarge," said Paddington gratefully. "It means I shan't have to speak to Sir Bernard Crumble after all. If you don't mind, I shall always come here first if ever my shopping basket on wheels gets towed away."

"That's what we're here for," said the sergeant. "Although I think I should warn you, it may be a bit heavier now than when you first set out this morning."

"Quite right too," said Paddington's friend Mr. Gruber when they eventually sat down to their elevenses and Paddington told him the full story, including the moment when he got back to the market and found to his surprise that his basket on wheels was full to the top with fruit and vegetables.

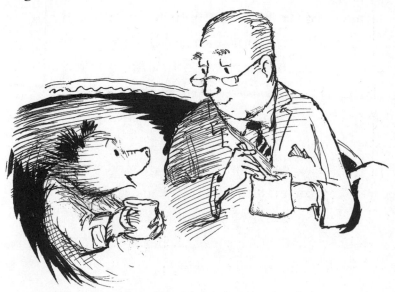

"You have been a very good customer over the years, and I daresay none of the traders want to see you go elsewhere. It is a great compliment to you, Mr. Brown.

"All the same," he continued, "it must have been a nasty experience while it lasted. If I were you, I would start your elevenses before the cocoa gets cold. You must be in need of it."

Paddington thought that was a very good idea indeed. "Perhaps," he said, looking up at the antique clock on the wall of the shop, "just this once, Mr. Gruber, we ought to call it twelveses."

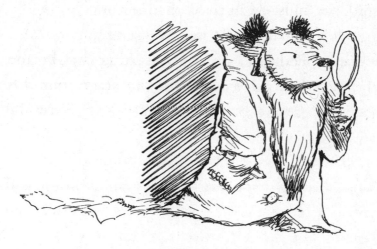

Chapter Two

PADDINGTON'S GOOD TURN

LIKE MOST HOUSEHOLDS up and down the country,
number 32 Windsor Gardens had its own set
routine.

In the case of the Brown family, Mr. Brown
usually went off to his office soon after breakfast,
leaving Mrs. Brown and Mrs. Bird to go about
their daily tasks. Most days, apart from the times

when Jonathan and Judy were home for the school holidays, Paddington spent the morning visiting his friend Mr. Gruber for cocoa and buns.

There were occasional upsets, of course, but on the whole the household was like an ocean liner. It steamed happily on its way, no matter what the weather.

So when Mrs. Bird returned home one day to what she fully expected to be an empty house and saw a strange face peering at her through the landing window, it took a moment or two to recover from the shock, and by then whoever it was had gone.

What made it far worse was the fact that she was halfway up the stairs to her bedroom at the time, which meant the face belonged to someone *outside* the house.

She hadn't seen any sign of a ladder on her way in; but all the same she rushed back downstairs again, grabbed the first weapon she could lay her hands on, and dashed out into the garden.

Apart from a passing cat, which gave a loud shriek and scuttled off with its tail between its legs when it caught sight of her umbrella, everything appeared to be normal, so it was a mystery and no mistake.

When they heard the news later that day, Mr. and Mrs. Brown couldn't help wondering if Mrs. Bird had been mistaken, but they didn't say so to her face in case she took umbrage.

"Perhaps it was a window cleaner gone to the wrong house," suggested Mr. Brown.

"In that case he made a very quick getaway," said Mrs. Bird. "I wouldn't fancy having him do our windows."

"I suppose it could have been a trick of the light," said Mrs. Brown.

Mrs. Bird gave one of her snorts.

"I know what I saw," she said darkly. "And whatever it was, or *who*ever it was, they were up to no good."

The Browns knew better than to argue, and Paddington, who had been given a detective outfit for his birthday, spent some time testing the windowsill for clues. Much to his disappointment, he couldn't find any marks on it other than his own.

All the same, he took some measurements and carefully wrote down the details in his notebook.

In an effort to restore calm, Mr. Brown rang the police, but they were unable to be of much help either.

"It sounds to me like the work of Gentleman Dan, the Drainpipe Man," said the officer who came to visit them. "They do say he's usually in the Bahamas at this time of the year, but he could be back earlier than usual if the weather's bad.

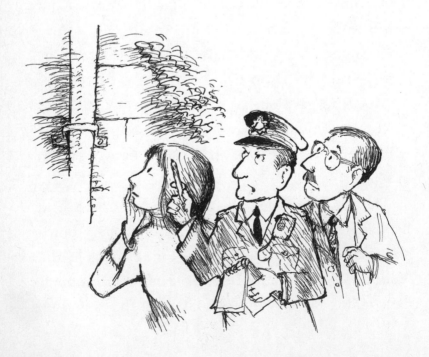

"He didn't get his name for nothing. He bides his time until he sees what he thinks are some empty premises, and then he shins up the nearest drainpipe. He can be in and out of a house like a flash of lightning. Never leaves any trace of what we in the force call his dabs, on account of the fact that being a perfect gentleman, he always wears gloves."

The Browns felt they had done all they could to allay Mrs. Bird's fears, but the officer left them with one final piece of advice.

"We shall be keeping a lookout in the area for the next few days," he said, "in case he strikes again. But if I were you, to be on the safe side I'd invest in a can of Miracle nondry antiburglar paint and give your downpipes a coat as soon as possible.

"It's available at all good do-it-yourself shops. Mark my words, you won't be troubled again, and if by any chance you are, the perpetrator will be so covered in black paint he won't get very far before we pick him up.

"Not only that," he said, addressing Mr. Brown before driving off in his squad car, "you may find you get a reduction on your insurance policy."

"It sounds as though he's got shares in the company," said Mr. Brown skeptically, as he followed his wife back indoors. "Either that or he has a spare-time job as one of their salesmen."

"Henry!" exclaimed Mrs. Brown.

In truth, the next day was Friday, and after a busy week at the office Mr. Brown had been looking forward to a quiet weekend. The thought of spending it up a ladder painting drainpipes was not high on his list of priorities.

In normal circumstances he might not have taken up Paddington's offer to help quite so readily.

"Are you sure it's wise?" asked Mrs. Brown when he told her. "It's all very well Paddington saying bears are good at painting, but he says that about a lot of things. Remember what happened when he decorated the spare room."

"That was years ago," said Mr. Brown. "Anyway, the fact that he ended up wallpapering over the door and couldn't find his way out again had nothing to do with the actual painting. Besides, it's not as if it's something we shall be looking at all the time. Even Paddington can't do much harm painting a drainpipe."

"I wouldn't be so sure," warned Mrs. Bird. "Besides, it isn't just one drainpipe. There are at least half a dozen dotted around the house. And don't forget, it's nondry paint. If that bear makes any mistakes, the marks will be there forever-more."

"There must come a time when it dries off," said Mr. Brown optimistically.

"We could get Mr. Briggs in," suggested Mrs. Brown, mentioning their local decorator. "He's always ready to oblige."

But Mr. Brown's mind was made up, and when he arrived back from his office that evening he brought with him a large can of paint and an assortment of brushes.

Paddington was very excited when he saw them, and he couldn't wait to get started.

That night he took the can of paint up to bed and read the small print on the side with the aid of a flashlight and the magnifying glass from his detective outfit.

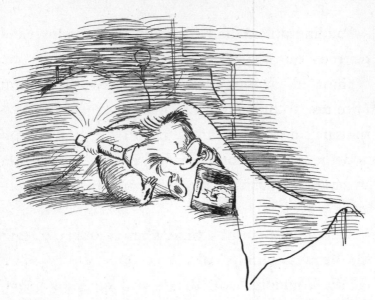

According to the instructions, a lot of burglars climbed drainpipes in order to break into people's homes. In fact, the more he read, the more Paddington began to wonder why he had never seen one before; it sounded as though the streets must be full of them. There was even a picture of one on the back of the tin. He looked very pleased with himself as he slid down a pipe, a sack over his shoulder bulging with things he had taken. There was even a thinks balloon attached to his head saying: "Don't you wish you had done something about *your* pipes?"

Paddington opened his bedroom window and peered outside, but luckily there were no drainpipes anywhere near it; otherwise he might have tested the paint there and then, just to be on the safe side.

Before going to sleep, he made out a list of all the other requirements, ready for the morning. Something with which to open the tin, a wire brush for cleaning the pipes before starting work, a pair of folding steps— the instructions suggested it was only necessary to paint the bottom half of the pipe; there was no need to go all the way up to the top—and some paint remover to clean the brushes afterward.

The following morning, as soon as breakfast was over, he waylaid Mrs. Bird in the kitchen and persuaded her to let him have some plastic gloves and an old apron.

Knowing who would be landed with the task of getting any paint stains off his duffle coat if things went wrong, the Brown's housekeeper was only too willing to oblige.

"Mind you, don't get any of that stuff on your whiskers," she warned, as he disappeared out through the back door armed with his list. "You don't want to spoil your elevenses."

Paddington's suggestion that it might be a good idea to have them *before* he started work fell on deaf ears, so he set to work gathering the things he needed from the garage. While he was there, he came across a special face mask to keep out paint fumes.

Clearly it wasn't meant for bears, because although it covered the end of his nose, it was nowhere near his eyes. All the same, having slipped the elastic bands over his ears to hold the mask in place, he spent some time looking at his reflection in the wing mirror of Mr. Brown's car, and as far as he could make out, all his whiskers were safely tucked away inside it.

Once in the garden, he set to work with a wire brush on a rainwater pipe at the rear of the house.

"I must say, he looks like some creature from outer space," said Mrs. Bird, gazing out of the kitchen window.

"At least it keeps him occupied," said Mrs. Brown. "I can't help being uneasy whenever he's at a loose end."

"The devil finds work for idle
paws," agreed Mrs. Bird, almost
immediately wishing she
hadn't said it in case she was
tempting fate.

But much to
everyone's surprise,
Paddington made
such a good job
of the first pipes

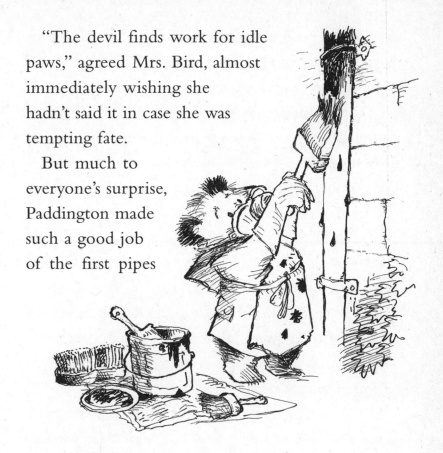

even Mrs. Bird's eagle eyes couldn't find anything
amiss when she inspected them. There wasn't a
single spot of paint to be seen anywhere on the
surrounding brickwork.

And even if it meant she would never be able to use
her rubber gloves or her apron again, she didn't have

the heart to complain. It was a small price to pay for having number 32 Windsor Gardens made secure, *and* keeping Paddington occupied into the bargain.

"What did I tell you, Mary?" said Mr. Brown, looking up from his morning paper when she passed on the news.

"I only hope he doesn't try shinning up the pipes to see if it works," said Mrs. Brown. "You know how keen he is on testing things."

"It's a bit like giving someone a hot plate and telling them not to touch it," agreed Mrs. Bird.

As it happened, similar thoughts had been going through Paddington's mind most of the morning. At one point when he stopped for a rest, he even toyed with the idea of hiding around a corner in the hope that Gentleman Dan might turn up, but with only one more drainpipe to go, he decided he'd better finish off the work as quickly as possible.

It was the one just outside the landing window at the side of the house, which had been the cause of all the trouble in the first place, and he had left it until last because he wanted to make an especially good job of it for Mrs. Bird's sake.

Having scrubbed the bottom section of the pipe clean with the wire brush, he mounted the steps and began work on the actual painting.

He hadn't been doing it for very long before he heard a familiar voice.

"What are you doing, bear?" barked Mr. Curry.

Paddington nearly fell off the steps with alarm. The last person he wanted to see was the Browns' next-door neighbor.

"I'm painting Mr. Brown's drainpipes," he announced, regaining his balance.

"I can see that," growled Mr. Curry suspiciously. "The thing is, bear, why are you doing it?"

"It's some special paint that never dries," said Paddington. "It's very good value."

"Paint that never dries?" repeated the Browns' neighbor. "It doesn't sound very good value to me."

"It was recommended to Mr. Brown by a

policeman," said Paddington importantly. "I've nearly finished all the pipes and I haven't used half the tin yet.

"Mrs. Bird saw a face at the window when she came home from her shopping the other day," he explained, seeing the skeptical look on Mr. Curry's face. "The policeman thought it might have been someone called Gentleman Dan, the Drainpipe Man, who climbed up this very pipe. Mrs. Bird said it gave her quite a turn. She hasn't got over it yet."

"I'm not surprised," said Mr. Curry. "Let's hope they catch him."

"I don't think he'll be back," said Paddington. "Not if he saw Mrs. Bird on the warpath, but Mr. Brown thinks it's better to be safe than sorry."

"Hmm," said Mr. Curry. "What did you say it's called, bear?"

"Miracle Nondry Paint for Outside Use," said Paddington, reading from the can. He held it up for Mr. Curry to see. "You can buy it in any good do-it-yourself shop."

"I don't want to do it myself, bear!" growled Mr. Curry. "I have more important things to do.

Besides, I'm on my way out."

He paused for a moment. "On the other hand, I would be more than interested in having my own pipes done. I do have some very valuable items about the house. Family heirlooms, you know."

"Have you really?" said Paddington with interest. "I don't think I've ever seen an heirloom before."

"And you're not starting with mine," said the Browns' neighbor shortly. "I don't have them on display for every Tom, Dick, and bear to see. I keep them tucked away—out of the sight of prying eyes."

Paddington couldn't help thinking, if that were the case, there was no point in the Browns' neighbor having his drainpipes painted, but Mr. Curry was notorious for being unable to resist getting something for nothing, even if it was something he didn't need.

A cunning look came over his face. "Did you say you have over half a tin of paint left?" he asked.

"Nearly," said Paddington. He was beginning to wish he hadn't mentioned it in the first place.

Mr. Curry felt in his trouser pocket. "Perhaps

you would like to have a go at my pipes while you're at it," he said. "I'm afraid I don't have very much change on me, but I could stretch to ten pence if you do a good job."

Paddington did a quick count-up on his paws. "Ten pence!" he exclaimed. "That's less than tuppence a pipe!"

"It's a well-known fact in business," said Mr. Curry, "that the bigger the quantity the less you pay for each individual item. It's what's known as giving discount."

"In that case," said Paddington hopefully, "perhaps I could do one of your pipes for five pence?"

"Ten pence for the lot," said Mr. Curry firmly. "That's my final offer. There's no point in having only one done."

"I think I'd better ask Mr. Brown if he minds first," said Paddington, clutching at straws. "It is his paint."

"Now, you don't want to do that, bear," said Mr. Curry, hastily changing his tune. "Let it be between ourselves."

Reaching into his pocket again, he lowered his

voice. "As I say, I have to go out now and I probably won't be back until this evening, so that will give you plenty of time to get it done. But if you make a really good job of it, I may give you a little extra. Here's something to be going on with."

Before Paddington had a chance to answer, something landed with a *plop* on the gravel at the foot of his steps.

Climbing down, he picked up the object and gazed at it for a moment or two before glancing up at Mr. Curry's house. Unlike the Browns' drainpipes, Mr. Curry's looked as though they hadn't seen a paintbrush in years. His heart sank as he turned the coin over in his paw. For a start, it didn't even look English. In fact, the more he thought about it, the 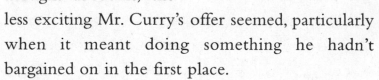 less exciting Mr. Curry's offer seemed, particularly when it meant doing something he hadn't bargained on in the first place.

While Paddington was considering the matter, he heard Mr. Curry's front door slam shut. It was followed almost immediately afterward by a clang from the front gate, and that in turn triggered off one of his brain waves.

Shortly afterward Paddington was hard at work again, and this time, knowing how cross the Browns would be on his behalf were they able to see what he was doing, he intended getting it over and done with as quickly as possible.

Later that day the Browns were in the middle of their afternoon tea when the peace was shattered by the sound of a violent commotion in the road outside their house.

At one point Mrs. Bird thought she heard loud cries of "Bear," and shortly afterward there was the sound of a police siren, but by the time she got to the front window all was quiet.

They had hardly settled down again before there was a ring at the front doorbell.

"I'll go this time, Mrs. Bird!" said Paddington eagerly, and before the others could stop him he was on his way.

When he returned, he was accompanied by the policeman who had visited them earlier in the week.

"Will someone please tell me what's going on?" said Mr. Brown.

"Allow me," said the officer before Paddington had a chance to open his mouth.

He produced his notebook. "First of all, a short while ago we received a call from one of your neighbors reporting a disturbance outside number thirty-three. We arrived at the scene as quickly as we could. The gate was wide open, and a gentleman covered in black paint was dancing about in the gutter shouting his head off. Assuming it must be Gentleman Dan, the Drainpipe Man, we placed him under immediate arrest.

"On our way back to the station, we managed to quiet him down"—the policeman looked up from his notebook—"which was no easy task, I can tell you. He informed us he was your next-door neighbor, so we removed the handcuffs and brought him back. I daresay you will be able to confirm you have a Mr. Curry living next door."

"I'm afraid we do," said Mrs. Brown.

"What did he look like?" asked Mr. Brown.

"Well, he's not exactly a bear lover, for a start," said the policeman. "Kept going on about the iniquities of someone called Paddington—"

"Say no more," broke in Mrs. Bird. "That's him."

"Well," continued the officer, "when we arrived back at his house, who should we meet coming out of the gate, but none other than Gentleman Dan, the Drainpipe Man. He must have seen us drive off and seized his chance. He had the cheek to say he'd gone to the wrong door by mistake."

"Did he get away with much?" asked Mr. Brown.

"Didn't have a thing on him," said the officer, "which is a pity, because I gather from Mr. Curry that he has a lot of valuable items, and we could have booked him on the spot.

"On the other hand, I don't think he'll be bothering us again for a while. Thanks to this young bear's efforts, we've not only got a picture of him, but we have his dabs for good measure."

He turned to Paddington. "I'd like to shake you by the paw for your sterling work," he said.

Paddington eyed the policeman's hand doubtfully. There was a large lump of something black attached to the palm.

"Perhaps you would like to borrow some of Mr. Brown's paint remover first," he said. "You won't want to get any of that on your steering wheel."

"You've got a point," said the policeman, taking a look at it himself. "Seeing as how I recommended it in the first place, I can't really complain, but . . ."

"I still don't quite understand," said Mr. Brown after the officer had left. "What's all this about painting Mr. Curry's front gate?"

Paddington took a deep breath. "I thought if I stopped any burglars from getting into his garden in the first place, they wouldn't be able to break into his house, and it would save using up all your paint on his downpipes. I forgot Mr. Curry still had to get back in!"

The Browns fell silent as they digested this latest piece of information.

"It seemed like a good idea at the time," said

Paddington lamely.

"You can't really blame Paddington, Henry," said Mrs. Brown. "You did take him up on his offer, after all."

"How much was Mr. Curry going to pay you for doing his pipes?" asked Mr. Brown.

"Ten pence," said Paddington

"In that case," said Mrs. Bird, amid general agreement, "I have no sympathy. That man deserves all he gets. *And* he knows it.

"If he says anything to you about it," she added grimly, turning to Paddington, "tell him to come and see me first."

"Thank you very much, Mrs. Bird," said Paddington gratefully. "If you like, I'll go around and tell him now."

The Browns exchanged glances. "It's very kind of you, Paddington," said Mrs. Brown. "But you've had a very busy day, and I do think it's a case of 'least said, soonest mended.' Why don't you put your paws up for a while?" Having considered the matter, Paddington thought it was a very good idea indeed. And funnily enough, Mr. Curry never did mention the day he *didn't* get his drainpipes painted, although for some weeks to come, whenever Paddington waved to the Browns' neighbor over the garden fence, he received some very black looks in return.

They were even darker than the color of his front gate, which now remained permanently open.

On the other hand, Mrs. Bird never again saw a face looking at her through the landing window.

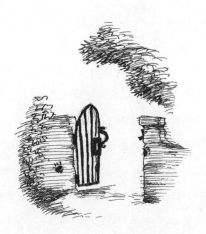

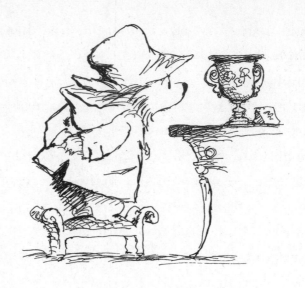

Chapter Three

PADDINGTON STRIKES A CHORD

PADDINGTON ALWAYS LOOKED forward to his morning chats with Mr. Gruber. One of the things that made visiting his friend's antique shop in the Portobello Road so special was the fact that it was never the same two days running. People came from far and wide to seek Mr. Gruber's advice. If it wasn't someone looking for an old painting or a bronze statue, it was someone else browsing through his vast collection of books, which covered practically every subject under the sun.

In time Paddington became quite knowledgeable about antiques himself; so much so, he could immediately tell a piece of genuine Spode china from an ordinary run-of-the-mill item of crockery, although he would never have dared pick any of it up in case he dropped it by mistake.

"Better safe than sorry" was Mr. Gruber's motto.

That apart, since both of them had begun life in a foreign country, they were never short of things to talk about.

During the summer months they often had their elevenses sitting in deck chairs on the pavement outside the shop, discussing problems of the day in peace and quiet before the crowds arrived.

Paddington couldn't help but notice his friend usually had a faraway look in his eyes whenever he spoke of his native Hungary.

"When I was a boy," Mr. Gruber would say, "people used to dance the night away to the sound of balalaikas. That doesn't seem to happen anymore."

Having been born in Darkest Peru, Paddington had no idea what a balalaika was, let alone what it sounded like, but with Mr. Gruber's help he did learn to play a tune called "Chopsticks" on an ancient piano at the back of the shop.

It wasn't easy, because having paws meant he often played several notes at the same time, but Mr. Gruber said anyone with half an ear for music would recognize it at once.

"Music is a wonderful thing, Mr. Brown," he was wont to say. "'Chopsticks' may not be top of what is known as the Pops, but if you are able to play it on the piano you will always be in demand at parties."

On cloudy days, when there was a chill in the air, they made a habit of retiring to an old horsehair sofa at the back of the shop, and it was on just such a morning, soon after his adventure with the shopping basket on wheels, that Paddington arrived rather earlier than usual and found to his surprise that Mr. Gruber had acquired a new piano.

It was standing in almost exactly the same spot as the old one had been: near the stove where his friend made the cocoa.

There was no sign of Mr. Gruber, which was most unusual, so to pass the time Paddington decided to have a go at playing what had become known as "his tune," when something very strange happened.

As he raised his paws to play the opening notes, the keys began going up and down all by themselves!

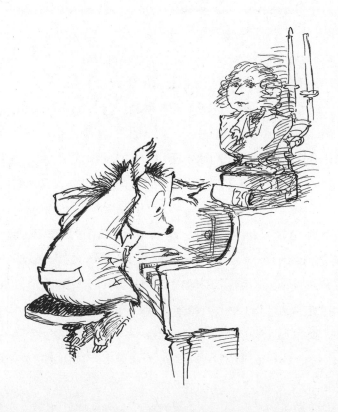

He had hardly finished rubbing his eyes in order to make sure he wasn't dreaming when he had yet another surprise. Out of the corner of his eye he saw Mr. Gruber crawl out from underneath a nearby table.

"Oh, dear," said Paddington, "I hope I haven't broken your new piano."

Mr. Gruber laughed. "Have no fear of that, Mr. Brown," he said. "It is what is known as a player piano, and it works by electricity. You don't see many around these days. I've just been plugging it in to make sure it works properly."

"I don't think I have ever seen a piano that plays a tune all by itself before," said Paddington. "We didn't have anything like that in Darkest Peru. But then, we didn't have electricity either," he added sadly.

While Mr. Gruber set about making the cocoa, Paddington took a closer look at the keyboard. It really was uncanny the way the keys went up and down in time to the music, and he tried following their movement with his paws without actually touching them. In the beginning he found it was hard to keep up with them, but after several goes it really began to look as though he was actually playing the tune.

"Look, Mr. Gruber," he called. "I can even do it cross paws!"

"I should watch out," warned his friend, looking up from the saucepan. "It's the 'Tritsch Tratsch Polka.' You will need to sit very tight."

But it was too late. Even as Mr. Gruber spoke, the music reached a crescendo and Paddington suddenly found himself lying on the floor with his legs in the air.

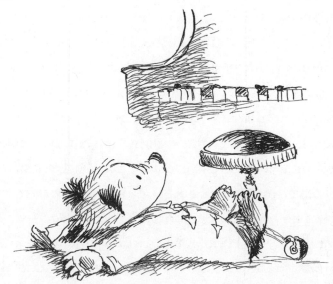

Mr. Gruber ran to switch the machine off. "I'm afraid it's a case of trying to run before you can walk, Mr. Brown," he said, helping Paddington to his feet. "I think perhaps you should try starting with something a little slower. I will see what I can find."

Opening the lid of a long cardboard box, he produced a roll of paper on a spindle, and unwinding it slightly, he held it up for Paddington to see.

Although he didn't say so, Paddington felt disappointed. It looked rather as if the moths had been at it.

"It seems to have a lot of holes in it," he said.

"Well spotted," said Mr. Gruber. "You have hit the nail on the head as usual, Mr. Brown. That is the secret behind a player piano. It works by blowing air through those holes as they go past. When the roll goes through at the correct speed, every time a hole passes a nozzle, the blast of air sets a lever in motion, and that in turn operates the correct note on the keyboard."

While he was talking, Mr. Gruber opened a small door above in the front of the piano, rewound the roll of paper already in there, and replaced it with the new one.

"It sounds very complicated," said Paddington, dusting himself down.

"It is really no more complicated than you or I picking up a mug of cocoa and drinking it," said Mr. Gruber. "When you think about it, that is also something of a miracle. I suggest we have our elevenses first, and then you can try out the tune I've just put in. It's Beethoven's *Moonlight Sonata*. I'm sure you will find it much easier."

It sounded like a very good idea, and Paddington hastily unpacked the morning supply of buns.

After they had finished the last of them and drained their mugs of cocoa, he climbed back on to the stool. This time, because the music was so much slower, he was even better at following the movement of the keys, and several passersby stopped outside the shop to watch.

"I wonder if Mr. Beethoven did a 'Chopsticks' roll?" he said. "I expect he would have been very good at playing that."

"I doubt it," said Mr. Gruber. "He was a very

famous composer, and he wouldn't have had the time. Besides, this machine wasn't invented until long after he died.

"If you close your eyes," he continued, "and sway gently with the music, I'm sure a great many people will think you really are playing it."

Following his friend's instructions, Paddington had another go, and by the time he reached the end of the piece, the pavement outside the shop was thronged with sightseers.

"Bravo!" said Mr. Gruber, joining in the applause as Paddington stood up and bowed to the audience. "What did I tell you, Mr. Brown? I think even Beethoven himself would have been taken in."

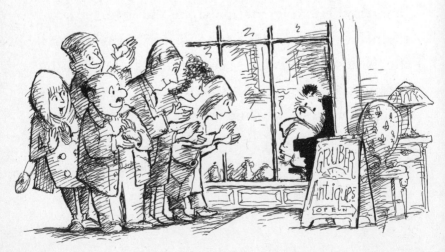

Shortly afterward, having thanked Mr. Gruber for the cocoa, Paddington bid him good-bye and made his way out of the shop, raising his hat to the crowd outside as he went. A number of people took his photograph, still more wanted his autograph, and several more dropped coins into his hat before he had a chance to put it back on. They felt quite cold when they landed on his head.

One way and another he was so excited he couldn't wait to tell the Browns all about it, so as soon as he was able to escape from the crowd of admirers, Paddington set off as fast as he could in the direction of Windsor Gardens.

He hadn't gone far before he realized he was being followed. In a strange way it wasn't unlike the player piano. Each time he put a foot down on the pavement, it was echoed by a footstep close behind him.

Looking back over his shoulder as he stopped at some traffic lights, he saw a figure wearing a long black overcoat and a fur hat waving at him.

"Stop! Stop!" called the man.

"This whole thing is quite extraordinary,"

continued the newcomer, removing a glove as he drew near. "I have never seen a bear play the piano before. Allow me to shake you by the, er . . . paw."

Paddington hastily wiped the nearest one on his duffle coat before holding it out.

"It's quite easy really," he began. "You see . . ."

"Ah, such modesty." The man glanced at Paddington's shopping basket on wheels. "I see you take your sheet music everywhere with you. How very wise."

"It isn't music," said Paddington. "It's Mrs. Bird's vegetables."

Reaching inside the basket, he took out a carrot and held it up for the other to see.

"Ah!" said the man, masking his disappointment. "It's good to see you haven't lost the common touch."

He pointed to a large poster on a nearby wall, one of many Paddington had recently seen dotted about the area. "I don't suppose for one moment you would care to do a recital for me, would you? I'm putting on a concert in aid of charity, and a piano-playing bear is just the kind of thing I need to round things off. The icing on the cake, as it were."

"Jonathan and Judy will be home for the half term, and Mr. Brown is taking us all to see it as a treat," said Paddington doubtfully. "So I shall be there anyway."

"Splendid!" exclaimed the man. "In fact, it couldn't be better."

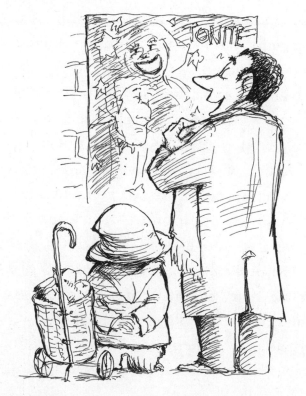

"I shall have to ask Mr. Gruber first," said Paddington. "It is his piano, and he says there aren't many like it left in the world."

"Leave all that to me," said the man. "Don't say another word. You shall have the best piano that money can buy. One that will suit your unique talents. Your obbligatos have to be heard to be believed. As for your glissandos . . . words fail me."

Paddington had no idea what the man was talking about, but he couldn't help feeling pleased. "It isn't easy with paws," he admitted. "I fell off the stool when I was playing the 'Trish Trash Polka.'"

"It happens to the best of players," said the man, brushing it aside. "Perhaps we had better have your paws insured. On the other hand, you may have been trying to run before you could walk."

Paddington stared at him. "It happened only this morning," he said excitedly. "And that's exactly what Mr. Gruber said."

He considered the matter for a moment or two. "I shall need some rolls," he announced.

"My dear sir"—the man raised his hands to high heaven—"you shall have all the rolls you need at the party afterward. They will be yours for the asking."

"It will be too late then," said Paddington. "I need them while I'm playing."

"You do?" The man looked at him in amazement.

"This is fantastic," he cried. "A novelty act! I can hardly believe my ears. There may be other bears in the world who play the piano, although I can't say I've come across any before, but there can't be many who have their supper at the same time."

"If you like," said Paddington eagerly, "I could eat a marmalade sandwich while I'm playing. I usually keep one under my hat in case of an emergency."

The man went into ecstasies at the thought.

"I can see it all," he cried, closing his eyes as he gazed heavenward. "You might save that until the end. It could bring down the house."

Paddington eyed him nervously. "I hope it doesn't land on me," he said.

"Ah, so you tell jokes as well," said the man. "This gets better and better."

Reaching into an inside pocket, he produced some papers. "May I have your signature, kind sir? I just happen to have a form in my pocket."

While he was talking, he handed Paddington a gold pen. "Just sign along the dotted line."

Paddington did his best to oblige, and because the man looked important, he added his special paw print to show it was genuine.

"Forgive my asking," said the man, eyeing the print with interest. "Are you by any chance Russian?"

"I was," said Paddington, "but I'm nearly home now."

His words fell on deaf ears as the man tried reading the writing above the blobs. "Is that where you were born . . . Paddington?"

"No," said Paddington. "It's my name. I've always been called that, ever since Mr. and Mrs. Brown found me in the railway station."

"In that case, we must change it to avoid any confusion," said the man. "We don't want the audience turning up at the wrong place, do we?"

"Change it!" repeated Paddington hotly.

"How about Padoffski?" said the man. "It will look better when I overstamp the posters, but you're not to tell anyone that."

"How about Mrs. Bird?" asked Paddington. "She doesn't like changes."

"Not until after the concert," said the man, tapping the side of his nose. "Let it be a surprise.

"Afterward," he said, "we must strike while the iron's hot and look to the future. What would you say to a world tour?"

"I wouldn't mind visiting the Home for Retired Bears in Lima," said Paddington. "It would be a nice surprise for Aunt Lucy."

"I don't normally do retirement homes," said the man. "More often than not the audience is fast asleep by the end of the program."

"I'm sure Aunt Lucy would poke them with her knitting needle if they were," said Paddington loyally.

"Mmm, yes." The man eyed him doubtfully. "We shall have to see. First things first. We need to think about your entrance on the night. It's a pity you can't come up through the floor, like cinema organs used to in the old days."

"I expect I could borrow Mr. Brown's saw," said Paddington eagerly.

"I must say, you're not short of ideas," said the man admiringly. "We shall make a very good team. Now that I am your manager, I can see it all."

"You are?" exclaimed Paddington, looking most surprised.

"Remember," said the man, holding the piece of paper aloft. "You signed along the dotted line. It's all down here in black and white.

"Do you happen to know Purcell's *Passing By*?" he continued before Paddington had a chance to reply.

"Is he really?" said Paddington, looking around. "I didn't see him."

"He is a famous composer," said the man. "And that's the name of a song he wrote. I thought I might include it in your program."

"I'll ask Mr. Gruber," said Paddington. "He's bound to know."

"I would rather you didn't," said the man. "In fact, I would much rather you didn't tell anyone."

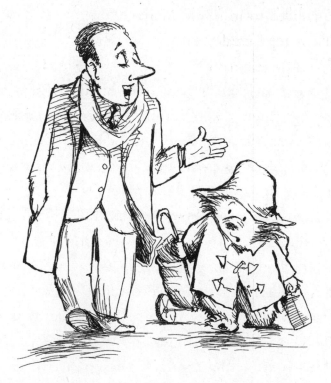

He tapped the side of his nose again. "Mum's the word."

"How about Mrs. Bird?" asked Paddington. "She's not a mum, and she knows everything."

"Especially Mrs. Bird by the sound of it," said the man. "Remember, walls have ears, and whatever else happens, we *must* keep it a secret until after the concert. Listen carefully and I will give you your instructions for the night."

"Wonders will never cease," said Mrs. Bird two mornings later. "Paddington's had a bath without being asked. He also wanted to know if I could get some stains off his duffle coat. He had a marmalade chunk stuck to one of the toggles."

"Oh, dear," said Mrs. Brown. "That *is* a bit worrying."

Having a bear about the house was a heavy responsibility, and there were times when it was hard to picture what was going on in Paddington's mind.

"He's been acting strangely these last two days," she said. "Ever since he got back from the market. He was going around peering at the walls this morning, and when I asked him if anything was the matter, all he said was 'Mum's the word.' Then he began tapping the side of his nose."

"I shouldn't worry too much," said Mrs. Bird. "There are no flies on that bear."

"I suppose that's why," said Mrs. Brown vaguely.

"I only hope he enjoys the concert tonight," said the Browns' housekeeper.

"Paddington enjoys anything new," said Mrs. Brown, trying to keep a brave face.

"That's one of the nice things about him. Henry thought it would be a treat."

It crossed Mrs. Bird's mind that since Mr. Brown went off to work every morning, he didn't have to face the consequences, but wisely she kept her thoughts to herself.

"We shall have to wait and see," she said.

In the event, however, even Mrs. Bird could hardly fault Paddington's behavior during the first half of the evening's performance. He even insisted on being at the end of the row when they took their seats.

"I expect he wants to be near the ice creams," whispered Jonathan.

Much to the Browns' relief, it didn't look as if the show involved any audience participation. It only needed a mind reader to ask for volunteers to go up onstage, or a magician who wanted to saw a member of the audience in two, and Paddington was usually the first to offer his services—almost always with disastrous results.

He didn't even embarrass them by eating one of his marmalade sandwiches during the interval.

"I'm saving it until later," he announced rather mysteriously.

The Browns heaved a sigh of relief. They still had vivid memories of the first time he had been taken to see a play. They had been occupying a box at the side the stalls, and Paddington had been so excited he accidentally dropped one of his sandwiches onto the head of a man sitting in a seat below them. At least they were safe from anything like that happening.

It wasn't until the show was nearing the end that Mr. Brown happened to glance along the row and realized Paddington was missing.

"Where can he have got to?" asked Mrs. Brown anxiously. "We shall never hear the last of it if he misses the grand finale. It's supposed to be something spectacular."

"Miss it, nothing!" exclaimed Jonathan, who had been sitting next to him. He pointed toward the stage as the curtain began to rise. "Look! He's in it!"

"Mercy me!" cried Mrs. Bird as she caught sight of a grand piano with a familiar figure seated at the keyboard. "Whatever is that bear up to now?"

Sporadic applause greeted the surprise item, particularly as it was some while before anything actually happened. Having spent some time staring at an area above the keys with a hopeful expression on his face, almost as though he expected to see a door of some kind, Paddington climbed off the stool and went around to the side of the piano.

Raising the lid as best he could, he peered inside.

But if he was hoping to find what he was looking for, he was clearly disappointed. After several loud twangs as he felt around with his paw, he closed the lid and disappeared underneath the piano.

Growing increasingly restive at the delay, certain sections of the audience began to boo, and there were one or two catcalls from rougher elements at the back of the hall.

When Paddington finally emerged, he was

mopping his brow, and there was a hunted look on his face as he called out to someone at the side of the stage.

"What did he say?" asked Mrs. Bird

"Something about not being able to find a socket," said Jonathan.

"'Chopsticks,' Mr. Brown!" came a loud voice from somewhere nearby. "'Chopsticks'!"

"Hear! Hear!" shouted someone else, or it could have been the same person disguising his voice.

Gradually the call was taken up by others until it seemed as though everyone was stamping their feet and shouting "Chopsticks" at the top of their voices.

As Paddington obliged, someone—it might have been the person who called out in the first place—led the audience in clapping to the beat of the music—and toward the end, when Paddington produced a sandwich from under his hat and took a large nibble, cheers shook the rafters.

The applause as Paddington stood to take his bow was deafening. So much so, he began looking anxiously at the ceiling.

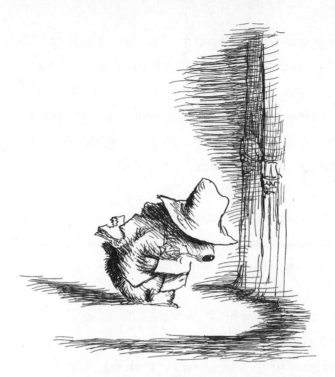

"Best turn I've seen in years," remarked a neighbor of the Browns as they left the theater. "We shall be seeing that bear's name in lights one of these days."

"If you want my advice," said Mr. Gruber with a twinkle in his eye when he bumped into them farther along the road, "I should retire at your peak, Mr. Brown. Otherwise, you may find the going downhill from now on."

Paddington stared at his friend. It really was uncanny how things kept repeating themselves.

"That's exactly what my manager said!" he exclaimed. "But he did tell me he's earmarked some of the money for the Home for Retired Bears in Lima. I must send Aunt Lucy a postcard and tell her to expect it."

Jonathan gave his sister a nudge. "I didn't know he had a manager. I wonder if that's who it was calling out for 'Chopsticks'?"

"He certainly saved the day," said Judy. "Have you any idea who it was, Mr. Gruber?"

But for some reason best known to himself, Paddington's friend was making haste to wave good night.

"To sum up," said Mrs. Bird, as they turned into Windsor Gardens and the familiar green front door of number 32 came into view, "it proves there's a lot of truth in the old saying 'A friend in need is a friend indeed.'"

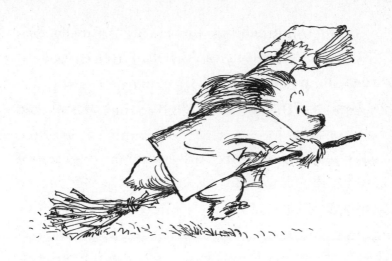

Chapter Four

Paddington Takes the Cake

One morning the Brown family was about to sit down to breakfast as usual when Mr. Brown noticed something strange going on in the garden.

"What *is* Paddington up to!" he said as a familiar figure in a duffle coat dashed past the French windows. "That's my best broom he's got hold of."

"Perhaps he's sweeping up," said Jonathan. "It

looks as though he's got a book of instructions."

"Even Paddington can't need instructions to sweep the patio," said Mr. Brown.

"Besides, it's my lawn broom. It's a special one made of twigs."

"Quick!" cried Judy as a shadowy figure shot past, heading back the way it had come. "There he goes again!"

From the brief glimpse they had, it looked as though Paddington was trying to keep the business end of Mr. Brown's broom between his legs with one paw while at the same time wave a book up and down with his other, not unlike a bird that had fallen out of its nest and was learning to fly.

A moment later there was a loud clatter from somewhere outside, and a dustbin lid rolled slowly past the French windows.

Jonathan jumped to his feet. "It sounds as though he's had a crash landing," he cried.

"Are you surprised?" asked Judy. "He had his eyes closed."

"It isn't like him to go rushing around the

garden before breakfast," broke in Mrs. Brown. "I do hope he's all right."

"He was as right as rain when he went to bed last night," said Judy. "I met him on the landing. He said he was going to do his accounts."

"Perhaps he found he was overdrawn," said Mr. Brown. "I'd better have a quiet word with him after breakfast."

Mrs. Bird gave a snort as she came into the room carrying a coffeepot. "There's nothing wrong with that bear's accounts," she said. "If you ask me, he's planning something. Earlier on he was asking me if I had any pumpkins."

"Ssh!" warned Mrs. Brown. "Here he comes."

The Browns were only just in time. They had scarcely settled down, trying to look as though butter wouldn't melt in their mouths, when Paddington entered the room.

After mopping his brow several times with a napkin, he joined them at the table, and while he was unscrewing the lid on the marmalade jar they managed to get a closer look at his book.

Most of the cover was filled with the silhouette

of an elderly lady astride a broomstick. The pointed hat she wore matched her sharply pointed nose as she hovered above a row of chimney pots. Far from being called *Teach Yourself to Fly*, the book bore the words *Everything You Need to Know About Witches, Warlocks, and Hobgoblins*.

Mr. Brown gave a groan. "Of course! It's October thirty-first."

"Halloween," said Judy.

"Trick-or-treat time," added Jonathan.

Paddington spread a liberal helping of marmalade on his freshly buttered toast.

"Mr. Gruber lent it to me," he explained. "I haven't read anything about warlocks or hobgoblins yet, but there's a very good chapter on witches and making masks. And there's another one telling you how to decorate a patio using lanterns made out of hollowed-out pumpkins. They're called jack-o'-lanterns, and if you put a lighted candle inside them it keeps evil spirits away.

"There's another chapter on superstitions," he continued. "It says if you take a three-legged stool and sit at some crossroads while the church clock strikes midnight, it will tell you the names of all those who will die during the next twelve months."

"Very cheering, I must say," said Mrs. Bird. "I know one thing. Anyone who sits on a stool near our crossroads at midnight could well end up at the top of the list."

All the same, Paddington's enthusiasm was infectious and as soon as the rest of the family finished their meal they gathered around his chair.

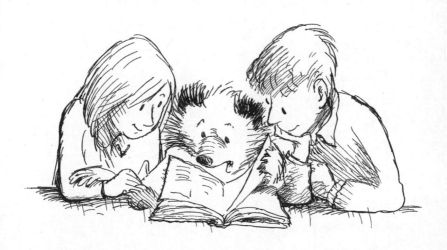

"I've never been to a Halloween party," he said wistfully. "I don't think they have them in Darkest Peru."

Mrs. Brown caught her husband's eye. "We haven't had one for ages, Henry," she said. "It might be fun."

"Please, Dad," chorused Jonathan and Judy.

Mr. Brown weakened. "Perhaps a small one," he said. "Just for the family, but no more. It's bad enough as it is with all those people ringing the front doorbell and calling 'Trick or treat' through the letter box. The only time I didn't answer it last year, we lost our dustbin lid."

"It did get found in the canal," said Jonathan.

"I'll get some chocolate bars in," said Mrs. Brown hastily. "They always go down well."

Paddington turned over the page. "There's a recipe for a witches' brew," he read.

"It's called stir fly, and it sounds very interesting."

"I think you must mean 'stir *fry*,' dear," said Mrs. Brown. "Unless, of course, it's a misprint."

Jonathan took a closer look. "No," he said firmly. "Paddington's right. It *is* stir *fly*."

"It gives the recipe," announced Paddington, reading from the book. "It's a mixture of toenail clippings, bats' blood, and dead flies."

"Charming," said Mr. Brown. "I can't wait!"

"They're not real," piped up Judy, seeing the look on everyone's faces. "You can make pretend toenail clippings out of pieces of chicory, and for the flies all you need are some old currants that have gone hard. Mix it all together with tomato ketchup, and Bob's your uncle."

"Bob's welcome to it, whoever he is," murmured Mr. Brown. "I'm not sure I wouldn't prefer the real thing."

"Look," said Jonathan, gazing over Paddington's shoulder. "There's something here about taking a kipper to bed with you."

"That's another very good chapter," said Paddington knowledgeably. "I read it under the eiderdown last night. It says if you take a kipper to bed and eat it before you go to sleep, the person you are going to marry will bring you a glass of water during the night to quench your thirst."

"Hmm," said Mrs. Bird. "I hope whoever it turns out to be is prepared to wash the sheets in the morning, that's all I can say."

"Anyway," said Judy, "you're not thinking of getting married, are you?"

"I might be," said Paddington darkly. "There is another way," he continued. "It says here, if you cut the letters of the alphabet out of some newspaper headlines and float them in a bowl of water, they will spell out the name for you."

Mr. Brown pointedly glanced at his watch and then reached for his morning paper. "I think it's time I went to the office," he said. "It's a bit early in the day for origami."

"What a bit of luck it's half term," said Jonathan after Mr. Brown had said his good-byes. "We can help get everything ready."

"If I were you, Paddington," said Mrs. Bird, "I'd get down to the market as soon as possible. Once people begin to realize what day it is, there could be a run on pumpkins." She reached for her handbag. "While you're there you can get a box of night-lights to go inside them."

"Don't forget we need some chicory for the toenails," called Judy.

Paddington made a note of it, and in no time at all he set off with his list, leaving Jonathan and Judy to start making the masks.

"Very wise," said Mrs. Bird approvingly when she saw what they were up to. "Speaking from experience, that bear and glue pots are best kept as far apart as possible. He can help me with the pumpkins when he gets back."

"You don't think Paddington was serious about getting married, do you?" asked Judy when she and Jonathan were on their own.

"I can't picture him carrying anyone over the threshold if that's what you mean," said Jonathan. "He'd be bound to drop them, or else get stuck halfway through the door; besides, he's got to find someone first."

"It's hard to picture anyone wanting to share kippers in bed with him," said Judy, reaching for the paint. "It would be a bad start to married life. I think we're fairly safe."

By the time Paddington got back from the market, they had both made so many masks it was hard to find anywhere to sit. Having tried his paw unsuccessfully at painting one while standing up, Jonathan suggested that Paddington might look in the garage for some old pieces of frayed rope so that he could make a wig for himself.

Mrs. Bird set to work hollowing out the pumpkins, and as soon as that job was done, having left Jonathan and Judy to put the night-lights inside them, she turned her attention to the cooking, leaving Paddington to look for some way of dying his wig black.

One way or another everyone was kept busy, but if the first half of the day passed quickly, waiting for it to get dark seemed to take forever.

In order to pass the time, Paddington retired to his bedroom to write some Halloween poems while he was trying out his costume.

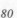

"I'm ready for the trick-or-treat part," he announced when he came back downstairs at long last.

With the addition of a black pointed hat similar to the one on the cover of Mr. Gruber's book, everyone agreed he made a very good witch indeed.

The finishing touch was a set of white fangs Judy had made for him out of some orange peel turned inside out.

"I wouldn't like to meet you on a dark night," said Jonathan when they went out into the front garden.

"I thought perhaps we could start with Mr. Curry, as he's nearest," said Paddington.

"Do you think that's wise?" asked Judy.

"I've written a special poem for him," said Paddington. "I don't want to waste it."

"You must like living dangerously," said Jonathan. "I doubt if you'll get anything out of him. It would be easier to get blood out of a stone."

"Pigs might fly!" agreed Judy.

"I don't suppose he'll recognize me in my outfit," said Paddington optimistically, as he set off through the front gate, leaving the others to hide behind the fence.

"I wouldn't bank on it," called Jonathan.

But he was too late, for Paddington was already out of earshot.

Having pressed Mr. Curry's bell push several

times, Paddington hid in the shadows, carefully keeping the lantern behind him so that his face wouldn't show.

"Yes?" barked the Browns' neighbor as he opened the door a fraction and peered through the gap. "Who is it?"

"Hurry, hurry, Mr. Curry," called Paddington, disguising his voice. "Give me a gift, and I'll be swift."

"Go away, bear!" exclaimed Mr. Curry. "How dare you! Any more of that nonsense and I shall call the police." And with that he slammed the door in Paddington's face.

"That settles it," said Jonathan when they heard what had happened. "It's time for tricks, not treats. I found a good one in your book while you were in the garage this morning. You tie one end of a length of cord to someone's front doorknob. Then you pull it tight and tie the other end to a convenient tree.

"After that you ring the front doorbell and hide. If it's done properly, when they try to open the door they think it's stuck. I've brought some cord in case it was needed."

"It'll serve him right for being so mean," said Judy.

"I'll do it," said Paddington eagerly. "Bears are good at knots."

He seemed so keen on the idea, the others didn't have the heart to say no. Instead, they kept watch while he hurried back to Mr. Curry's house armed with the cord.

Tying it to the doorknob took rather longer than he had bargained for, especially as he was trying to do it as quietly as possible, and it wasn't until he looked around for something he could tie the other end to that he realized Mr. Curry's front garden was like the proverbial desert. There wasn't a sign of a convenient shrub, let alone a tree.

Paddington was about to go back home and ask Jonathan's advice when the door suddenly opened.

"Who's that rattling my letter box?" barked Mr. Curry.

"I might have known!" he growled when he caught sight of Paddington hiding behind his pumpkin. "Up to your tricks again, bear?"

"Oh, no," said Paddington hastily. "They're not *my* tricks, Mr. Curry. They're in Mr. Gruber's book . . . I mean . . ."

The Browns' neighbor stared at him suspiciously. "What's that in your paw?" he demanded.

"It's my jack-o'-lantern," explained Paddington. He held the pumpkin up for Mr. Curry to see. "It's supposed to frighten off evil spirits, but it doesn't seem to be working very well—" He broke off as he caught sight of the look on the other's face.

"I meant, what's in your *other* paw?" barked Mr. Curry. "The one behind your back." And before Paddington could stop him, he had grabbed hold of the cord.

"I wouldn't pull it if I were you, Mr. Curry," said Paddington anxiously.

"Nonsense!" barked the Browns' neighbor. "There's only one way to find out where something goes; that's to give it a good tug." And without further ado he wound the cord around his other hand and pulled.

There was a loud bang as his door slammed shut. It was followed almost immediately by a sound of tinkling as a metal object landed on the path at their feet.

Mr. Curry stared at it. "That looks like a doorknob," he growled. "Have you any idea how it got there, bear? It might have caused a nasty accident."

Paddington held out his lantern and took a closer look. "I don't think it's one of ours, Mr. Curry," he said. "Mrs. Bird always keeps our doorknobs polished."

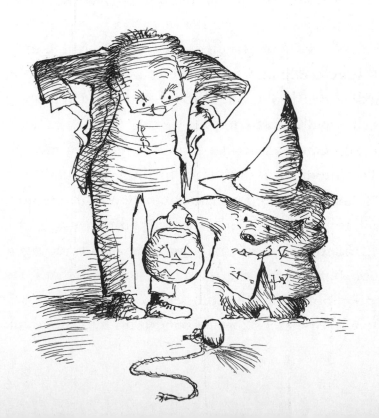

"That still doesn't explain what it's doing there," growled Mr. Curry.

"I was looking for a convenient tree," explained Paddington.

"I don't have any trees," growled Mr. Curry. "Nasty, untidy things, dropping their leaves everywhere."

"I know," said Paddington unhappily. "That's why the doorknob trick didn't work properly. Yours must have fallen off by mistake. It wasn't meant to."

"I'll give you tricks, bear," barked Mr. Curry. "They ought not to be allowed. If I had my way I'd—" He broke off. "Would you mind repeating what you've just said?"

Mr. Curry's face had grown purple with rage. In fact, Paddington didn't like the look of it at all, and he hastily lowered his lantern to be on the safe side.

"If you don't mind," he said, "I'd rather not."

But the Browns' neighbor was already doing it for him. "Are you trying to tell me that's *my* doorknob, bear?" he spluttered.

Clearly hardly able to believe his eyes, let alone

his ears, he gazed at his front door, then looked at the end of the cord tied around the knob.

"Do you realize," he bellowed, "you have locked me out of my own house?"

"No, Mr. Curry," said Paddington, glad to be on firm ground at last. "*I* didn't lock you out. You did it yourself. It's what Mrs. Bird calls a self-inflicted wound. She often says you're very good at those."

Raising his hat politely, he looked anxiously over his shoulder, but Jonathan and Judy were too well hidden to be of any help. "I think perhaps I'd better go now," he said. "We're having a Halloween party, and I don't want to be late."

Mr. Curry paused from whatever it was he had been about to say, and a cunning gleam came into his eyes. "Is that so, bear?" he said. "I thought I saw you doing a lot of coming and going this morning."

"There was a lot to get ready," said Paddington, only too pleased to change the subject. "Mrs. Bird's been very busy, baking cakes and making some special stir fly mixture."

"Seeing as I have been locked out of my house,"

said Mr. Curry, "it couldn't have happened at a better time. It's very kind of you to invite me, bear. Unless, of course," he added meaningly, "you would rather I told the Browns what you've just done."

Jonathan stood up. "That's torn it!" he said gloomily, overhearing the conversation. "Wait until Dad hears what's happened. He won't be pleased. Mr. Curry is the last person he'll want to see when he gets home."

"Paddington wasn't joking when he said bears are good at knots," agreed Judy. "How's he going to get out of this one?"

"I bet he finds a way," said Jonathan loyally. "He usually comes out on top."

Mr. Curry gazed around the Browns' living room as he made himself comfortable in Mr. Brown's favorite armchair. Having helped himself liberally from a bowl of chocolates, he gave a shiver and then stood up again.

"I think I'll move nearer the fire," he said. "I got cold standing outside."

Much to everyone's dismay he looked all set for

the rest of the evening.

"Now, bear," he said, addressing Paddington. "It's my turn. Seeing as you have kindly invited me to your party, I have a poem for *you*.

"You mentioned something just now about having some stir fry . . . so first of all, trick or treat, give me some of that to eat!"

Mrs. Bird pursed her lips, but before she had time to say anything Paddington jumped to his feet. "Don't worry, Mrs. Bird," he called, as he hurried out of the room. "Leave it to me."

It wasn't long before he returned carrying a large bowl and a spoon on a tray.

Mr. Curry scooped up the last of the chocolates and placed them inside his jacket pocket before turning his attention to Paddington's offering.

"You cannot say I do not try," said Paddington. "I'll give it to you, then I must fly."

"Thank you, bear," said Mr. Curry, licking his lips. And without further ado, he grabbed the spoon and began attacking the bowl.

Paddington waited until the Browns' neighbor had finished his second mouthful and was visibly slowing down. "I'm afraid it's a bit chewy," he said. "It's a special Halloween recipe."

"Most unusual," said Mr. Curry. "I've never had anything quite like it before. Aren't you having any, bear?"

"I don't think so, Mr. Curry," said Paddington. "Thank you very much. My Aunt Lucy always told me never to swallow flies. It's a bit difficult in Darkest Peru. They have a lot of them there. She had to keep her jars covered whenever she was making marmalade in case some went in. They're supposed to make you go thin."

Mr. Curry gave a snort. "Nonsense!" he barked. "That's an old wives' tale if ever I heard one. Besides, what's that got to do with—?" He broke off, the spoon halfway to his mouth. "Why are you telling me that, bear?"

"I thought you might be interested," said Paddington innocently. "I did give your bowl a good stir before I brought it in."

Mr. Curry jumped to his feet. "Bear!" he bellowed.

"Are you trying to tell me I've been eating . . . stirred *flies*?"

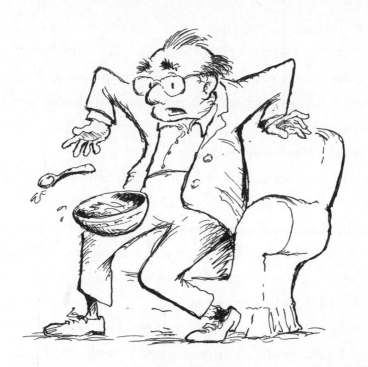

"May I get you another helping?" asked Mrs. Bird sweetly before Paddington had a chance to answer.

"No, you may not!" spluttered Mr. Curry. Clutching his stomach, he gave a loud groan. "That's the very last time I accept an invitation to one of your parties, bear!"

"Could we have that in writing?" murmured Jonathan, fortunately not loud enough for anyone other than Judy to hear.

"Accept an invitation indeed!" said Mrs. Bird. "I heard you browbeating Paddington just now. As for being locked out of your house, you know very well we keep a spare key for you in case of an emergency. Come with me."

And while Paddington took the remains of Mr. Curry's soup into the kitchen, Mrs. Bird led their uninvited guest into the hall.

Moments later, for the second time that evening the sound of a front door being slammed echoed around Windsor Gardens.

"Who would have believed it?" said Mrs. Brown.

"I told you Paddington would find a way," said Jonathan.

"Still waters run deep," said Judy.

"There's nothing still about that bear's waters," said Mrs. Bird as she came back into the room. "If you ask me, there's a lot goes on under that hat we don't know about."

"Would anyone else like any stirred flies?" she asked. "Or would you prefer pumpkin soup? I made it specially. You can't make lanterns without having a lot of the inside fruit left over."

"It's very good," said Paddington, licking his lips as he arrived back from the kitchen. "I've just been testing it."

"In that case," said Mr. Brown. "Come on, everyone. It's party time!"

Afterward they all voted it was the best soup they'd had in a long time.

"Aren't you going to take your hat off, Paddington?" asked Mrs. Brown when it was time to go to bed.

"If you don't," said Mrs. Bird, "the glue may melt during the night, then you'll be stuck with it."

Paddington considered the matter for a moment or two before he went upstairs. He felt very torn. "I suppose I'd better," he said at long last. "Otherwise I shan't be able to raise it if I meet someone I know when I'm out shopping. But if you don't mind, I'll take my lantern with me while the night-light is still burning. It's been such a nice Halloween I don't want to miss a minute of it."

"I know I've said it before," said Mrs. Bird as Paddington disappeared up the stairs, "but I'll say it again. That bear takes the cake!"

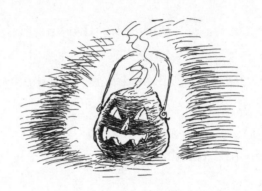

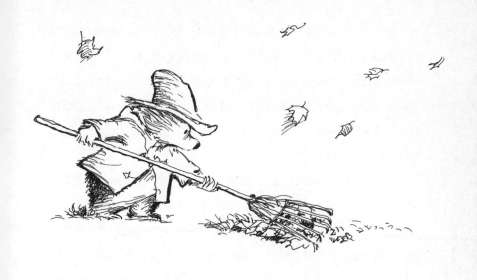

Chapter Five

PADDINGTON SPILLS THE BEANS

ONE BRIGHT DECEMBER morning Paddington decided to make himself useful in the garden. With Christmas not far away, he was anxious to earn some extra pocket money, so he set to work at the front of the house, clearing up the last of the autumn leaves and generally tidying up the flower beds.

He didn't want a repeat of the previous year's debacle, when he gave everyone in the family a diary he'd come across in a stall at the market. Like most bears, he had an eye for a bargain, and at the time five for the price of one sounded very good value indeed.

It wasn't until halfway through Boxing Day afternoon, when Mr. Brown laid down his pen at long last, having finished the arduous task of transferring all the names and addresses and birthday reminders from his old diary into the new one, that he happened to glance at the date and discovered the two were identical.

Having swept the leaves into a tidy pile, Paddington took some pruning shears out of his duffle coat pocket and turned his attention to the rosebushes in case they needed a final prune before winter set in.

A quick glance decided him against it. The roses were Mr. Brown's pride and joy, and he went to great pains to ensure they were pruned close to an outward facing bud.

Whenever Paddington looked at them, the only

buds he could find always seemed to face the wrong way, and that day was no exception.

He was in the middle of taking a closer look at one of the stems through his magnifying glass when he heard a cough. Looking around, he realized he was being watched.

"Ahem," said a man looking over the railing. "Please forgive me. I can see you're busy. Please don't bother to stand up."

Paddington looked most offended. "I *am* standing up," he announced.

"Oh!" The newcomer sounded rather flustered. "I do beg your pardon, but I assumed you were a jobbing gardener, a refugee from some foreign clime, perhaps? I wonder . . . are your employers at home?"

"My *employers*!" repeated Paddington, growing more and more upset. "But I *live* here. I'm trying to make my ends meet in time for Christmas. I was looking for some outward–facing buds, but I can't find any."

"I know just how you feel," said the man sympathetically.

He held up a clipboard. "I'm trying to conduct a survey, but so far I haven't found a single person to interview. Everybody in the road seems to be out."

"I expect it's because of your board," said Paddington knowledgeably. "Mrs. Bird says she never opens the door to a man with a clipboard. It usually means he's after something."

"Ah!" The man gave a hollow laugh. "Thank you very much for the tip. I'm not used to this kind of work, you see, and . . ." His voice trailed away under Paddington's gaze.

"Since you live here," he continued, "perhaps you wouldn't mind answering a few simple questions. It will only take up a minute or two of your valuable time. We are asking people about their views."

"I have a very good one from my bedroom window," said Paddington, only too happy to oblige. "On a clear day I can see the British Telecom Tower."

The interviewer allowed himself a smile. "How very interesting." He took a closer look at

Paddington. "Forgive my mentioning it, but from your accent I take it you are not . . . well . . . I mean, where exactly are you from?"

"Peru," said Paddington. "*Darkest* Peru."

"Darkest Peru?" repeated the man. "I've come across a good many Bulgarians and Poles coming over here to work, but I've never met anyone from Darkest Peru before." He consulted a sheet of paper on his clipboard. "There isn't even a box I can tick. If you don't mind my saying so, I hope there isn't a flood this winter."

"Mr. Curry had one last year," said Paddington.

"He did?" exclaimed the man excitedly. He jotted the name down. "Perhaps you could give me his address. I'll see if I can jog his memory."

"I would rather you didn't," said Paddington anxiously. "He's our next-door neighbor and we don't get on very well."

"Oh, dear," said the man. "Does it bring back unhappy memories for you?"

"No," said Paddington. "But it does for Mr. Curry. He had a burst pipe in his bathroom, and I was helping him mend it.

"He gave me a hammer to hold and told me that when he nodded his head I was to hit it. So I did. I didn't realize he meant the pipe."

"I see the problem," agreed the man. "It's not something you would forget in a hurry."

He turned over the page. "Changing the subject, do you have any complaints about the way you have been treated since you arrived in this country?"

Paddington considered the matter for a moment. "Well, it wasn't Mrs. Bird's fault," he said, "but my boiled egg was a bit runny this morning."

"Your boiled egg was a bit runny?" The man had started to write something down, but he crossed it out. "I hardly think that's a reasonable cause for complaint."

"It is if you're a bear," said Paddington hotly. "If you're a bear and the yolk dries on your whiskers, it makes them stick together and it's very painful. It hurts every time you open your mouth."

"Er, yes," said the interviewer, "I suppose it would. Did you register a complaint?"

Paddington looked taken aback at the thought.

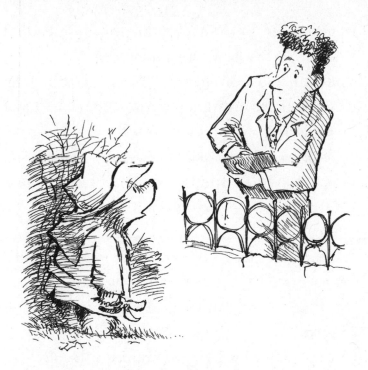

"I wouldn't dare," he said. "Mrs. Bird rules the house with a rod of iron."

"Really?" The man looked around nervously. "Does she carry it with her?"

"Oh, it's only a pretend one," said Paddington. "But she can be a bit fierce at times. Mr. Brown says that deep down she has a heart of gold. Anyway, she's out with Mrs. Brown doing the Christmas shopping, and both Jonathan and Judy are away at school. They're not due home until tomorrow, so I've been left in charge."

The man looked relieved. "This Mrs. Bird," he said. "I would like to know more about her. Do I take it she isn't a very good cook?"

"*Not a very good cook*?" repeated Paddington indignantly. "Mrs. Bird's dumplings are the best I've ever tasted. They're well known in the neighborhood."

"Dumplings well known in neighborhood," repeated the man, making an entry on his form.

"So is her marmalade," said Paddington. "It's full of chunks."

Feeling under his hat, he produced a sandwich. "You can try this one if you like. I made it myself the week before last."

It looked somewhat the worse for wear, and the man eyed it doubtfully. "I think I would rather not," he said.

"I always keep one under my hat in case of an emergency," explained Paddington, "but nothing's gone wrong for several weeks now."

"I don't suppose you happen to keep one of Mrs.

Bird's dumplings under there as well, do you?" asked the man. "I could take a picture of it on my mobile phone."

"A *dumpling!*" exclaimed Paddington. "Under my hat!" He gave the interviewer a very hard stare indeed.

The man's voice trailed away as he caught the look on Paddington's face. "May I ask how you got here in the first place?" he inquired, hurriedly changing the subject.

"I came in a small boat," said Paddington. "I was a stowaway."

"All the way from Darkest Peru?" The interviewer raised his eyebrows. "I know a lot of you boat people are desperate, but that sounds like a world record to me. Your paws must have been sore after all that rowing."

"Oh, I didn't have to row," said Paddington. "The boat was fixed to the side of a big ship. It was my Aunt Lucy's idea. I was a stowaway."

"All the same," said the man, "it can't have been easy."

"It certainly wasn't in the Bay of Biscuits," said

Paddington. "I had a job to stand up. The sea was so rough I nearly got washed overboard several times."

"Surely you mean the Bay of Biscay?" said the man.

"I called it the Bay of Biscuits," said Paddington firmly. "Someone was hanging over the ship's rail and they let go of a Garibaldi biscuit by mistake. It landed on my head, so I had it for dinner. I felt much better afterward."

"How many *B*s are there in 'Garibaldi'?" asked the man as he wrote it down.

"There aren't bees in a Garibaldi," said Paddington. "They have currants instead."

Taking a deep breath, the interviewer reached for his eraser. "This Aunt Lucy of yours," he continued. "Can you tell me more about her?"

"Well," said Paddington, "she's very wise. If it wasn't for her, I wouldn't be here at all. Besides, she taught me all I know. "

"Perhaps you could let me have her address," said the man. "I'd like to take her on board and make her part of my team. She sounds like just the kind of person we're looking for."

"I don't think that would be very easy," said Paddington. "She's living in the Home for Retired Bears in Lima. Besides, she doesn't play any ball games."

The interviewer gave Paddington a glassy stare as he reached for his eraser again.

"I had a clean form when I started out this morning," he said plaintively. "Now look at it!

"I suppose," he continued, trying another tack, "since your Aunt Lucy is in a home, she's . . . er . . . I mean, is there an uncle by any chance?"

"Oh, yes," said Paddington. "Uncle Pastuzo. But we haven't seen him since the earthquake."

"You mean you're an earthquake victim?" The man's pen fairly raced across the page. "Tell me more."

"Well," said Paddington, "there's not much to tell. I was fast asleep in a tree at the time. There was a loud rumble, and the earth began to shake. When I woke up everything looked different. Everyone else apart from Aunt Lucy had disappeared."

"Even your Uncle Pastuzo?" said the interviewer.

"Especially Uncle Pastuzo," said Paddington. "I think he must have known it was going to happen, because he went out early that day. But he left his old hat and a suitcase with a secret compartment behind, along with a note to say I could have them if anything happened to him."

"And you have never heard any more of him since?"

Paddington shook his head sadly. "That's why Aunt Lucy brought me up. She taught me my tables, and she taught me to say 'please' and 'thank you' when I'm out shopping and to raise my hat whenever I meet someone I know.

"She also taught me to count my blessings when things look black. It's the first thing she does when she wakes in the morning. She says nine times out of ten you have more than you think you have."

"Would that there were more about like her," said the man. He turned the page. "One last thing before I leave you in peace. What are your feelings about being a blood donor?"

"No thank you," said Paddington firmly. "I haven't had my elevenses yet and it might make me go wibbly woo."

"I shouldn't let that worry you," said the man. "You can lie down afterward, *and* they give you a nice cup of tea in the bargain."

"I prefer cocoa," said Paddington. "Bears do, you know."

"No, I didn't know that," said the man, entering the information on his form.

"While we are on the subject of medical matters," he continued, "if you don't fancy being a blood donor, how about donating one of your organs when the time comes?"

Paddington considered the matter for a moment or two. He wondered if he ought to mention Jonathan's mouth organ. It had been a nine days' wonder at the time, and everybody had breathed a sigh of relief when he took it back to school with him after the holidays.

"I don't have any myself," he said.

The man concealed a smile. "Oh, but you must have," he said. "Everyone has organs."

"Mr. Curry doesn't, for a start," said Paddington.

"Oh, dear," said the interviewer. "Poor man.

What with that *and* having his pipes frozen, he must be in a terrible state. I daresay he has to be tended day and night."

Paddington looked over his shoulder. "I don't think so," he said, lowering his voice. "He lives all by himself."

The man followed the direction of Paddington's gaze. "It gets worse and worse," he said. "Is that why the curtains are drawn?"

"Mrs. Bird says it's because he doesn't like people spying on him," said Paddington.

"I'm not surprised," said the man, "if he has no organs."

"Jonathan had one once," said Paddington. "But he swapped it with a boy at school for a pencil box."

The interviewer's eyes nearly popped out of their sockets. "Jonathan swapped one of his organs for a pencil box?" he repeated. "Do you know which one it was?"

"I don't know the name," said Paddington. "But it was very special. It had two tiers. One for ordinary pencils and another one for crayons."

"I don't mean the pencil box," said the man. "I mean which organ. This could be headline news! It's just the kind of material my editor is looking for."

"Oh, dear!" Paddington suddenly wondered if he had said the right thing.

"Are you absolutely certain you don't want to set an example?" said the man. "I wasn't meaning today, of course. It won't happen until after you . . ." He shifted uneasily underneath Paddington's hard stare. "Well, you know . . . after you er, um."

"After I er, um?" repeated Paddington.

"That's right," said the man. "It happens to us all at some time."

"It hasn't happened to me yet," said Paddington.

"I can see that," said the man, looking as though he was beginning to wish it had.

"One last thing," he remarked casually. "Can you tell me the name of Jonathan's school?"

"I'm very sorry," said Paddington, raising his hat politely to show the conversation was at an end. "I'm afraid I can't."

"What's it worth?" asked the interviewer. Taking

out his wallet, he fingered some notes.

"More than all the tea in China," said Paddington, remembering one of Mrs. Bird's favorite phrases.

"And if this doesn't work?" asked the man, detaching one of the notes, crackling it enticingly between his thumb and forefinger.

"I have a secret weapon," said Paddington. "I'll show you if you like."

Looking around to make sure nobody was watching, he gave the interviewer one of his hardest stares ever.

The man shuddered as though he had been struck by lightning, and something fell to the ground.

"That's another thing Aunt Lucy taught me," said Paddington. "It comes in very useful at times!"

"I think I might call it a day," said the man, hastily retrieving his pen. He handed the note across the railing. "You'd better have this anyway. It may help you to make your ends meet before Christmas.

"We're giving them away this week," he added.

"It's a thank-you present."

And with that he turned on his heels and disappeared down Windsor Gardens as though he had a train to catch.

Paddington gazed at the note for a moment or two. It didn't look like any sort of money he had seen before. Instead of the pound sign, there was a picture of an airplane, followed by a lot of words in small print. None of them seemed to make any sense, so he slipped it into his duffle coat pocket for safekeeping and hurried back into the house in case anyone else came along wanting to interview him.

"What do you think 'er, ums' are?" asked Mr. Brown.

It was the following day, and he had just arrived back from the station, having collected Jonathan and Judy, who were home for the Christmas holiday.

"You've been reading Paddington's postcard, Henry," said Mrs. Brown accusingly.

"I couldn't help it," said Mr. Brown. "It was lying on the hall table ready to be posted. Anyway, it sounds as though you've read it too."

"It's addressed to his Aunt Lucy," said Mrs. Brown. "I have no idea what it means, but he told her not to worry."

"If you ask me," said Mrs. Bird, "a spoonful of castor oil might not come amiss."

"Poor old Paddington," said Judy.

"Worse things happen at sea," said Jonathan cheerfully.

"I don't know about that," said Mr. Brown. "Look at this headline!"

He held up the front page of a local newspaper.

ORGAN REPLACEMENT SCANDAL
ROCKS LONDON'S WEST END

"I can't say I've felt any tremors," said Mrs. Bird, reading it out loud.

"I don't know where they get all these stories from in the first place," agreed Mrs. Brown. "I can't believe half of them are true. It doesn't sound like anywhere around here, thank goodness!"

"I wouldn't be too sure," warned Mr. Brown. "It's the same post code as ours—W11."

He continued reading. "'Where will it all end?'

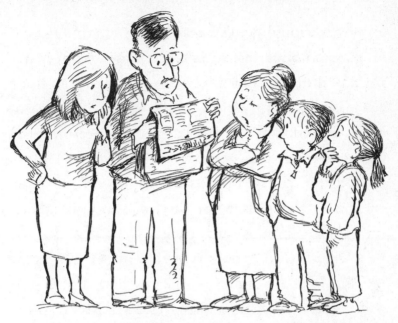

asks our man on the spot. Posing as an interviewer, our intrepid reporter Mervyn Doom managed to infiltrate the gang and obtain in-depth information from one of its hammer-carrying members.'"

"He makes it sound like some kind of ball game," interrupted Mrs. Brown. "Where on earth did you get the paper?"

"In Paddington station while I was waiting for the train," said Mr. Brown.

"Apparently the person he interviewed was disguised as a jobbing gardener. He gave the game away by saying he was looking for some outward-facing rose buds, not realizing it was long past the normal pruning season."

He looked up from the paper. "Can you imagine? It shows the type of person the authorities are up against.

"During the course of the interview our informant also let slip the fact that an undercover trade in organ transplants is rife.

"A local schoolboy swapped one of his for a pencil box—the name of the boy and the school have been withheld for legal reasons. Meanwhile, in this outwardly respectable neighborhood, others—bereft of everything that makes them tick—lie behind drawn curtains waiting for help."

"What *is* the world coming to?" exclaimed Mrs. Bird.

"And another thing," continued Mr. Brown, "according to this paper, the gates are about to open on a flood of boat people from Peru.

"Our question is, WHEN WILL SOMETHING BE DONE ABOUT IT? THERE IS NO TIME TO BE LOST!"

"Does it say who's behind it?" asked Mrs. Brown.

"Apparently the gang-master-in-chief is a woman," said Mr. Brown. "Notorious for her dumplings, and wielding an iron bar, she so terrifies those around her that the subject of the interview is forced to hide his marmalade sandwiches under his hat."

The Browns looked at one another. Suddenly it was all starting to sound much closer to home than they had thought.

"You don't think . . ." began Mr. Brown.

"Oh, dear, Henry," said Mrs. Brown. "I'm very much afraid I do."

"He asked if he could borrow your pruning shears yesterday morning," said Mrs. Bird.

"He wanted to do some work in the front garden."

"Don't tell me he was having a go at my roses?" exclaimed Mr. Brown, the full seriousness of the situation suddenly coming home to him.

"I don't like the sound of that last bit," said Mrs. Bird. "If the powers that be get hold of the story, there's no knowing what will happen. We can await the ring on the front doorbell."

The Browns exchanged anxious glances. In the beginning Paddington had just sort of happened, but over the years he had become so much a part of the family they couldn't picture life without him. They had certainly never thought of him as being a refugee, still less the possibility of his being an illegal one.

"I think they've starting doing something about things already," said Jonathan. "I saw an ambulance outside Mr. Curry's house soon after we got back. There was a terrible row going on. They were trying to tie him onto a stretcher."

"I suppose they might declare Paddington persona non grata," said Mr. Brown.

"That means an unwelcome person," said Judy, for her brother's benefit.

"Thanks a heap!" said Jonathan. "Who got an A Star in his exams?"

"Anyway," said Judy. "He's not a person. He's a bear."

"*And* he's always welcome," chimed in Mrs. Bird. "If anyone tries to take him away after all this time, they'll have me to deal with."

"Who in the world would want to report him?" asked Judy.

"I imagine Mr. Curry, for a start," said Jonathan, "if Paddington had anything to do with what happened this morning. Perhaps we could hide him under the floorboards—like the French did with escaped prisoners during World War Two."

"I shall never go out and leave that bear alone again," said Mrs. Bird.

"I'm sure he meant well," said Mrs. Brown.

"They can't," said Judy. "Take him away, I mean."

"There's no such word in the English language as 'can't,'" said Mrs. Bird grimly.

"What shall we tell Paddington?" broke in Mr. Brown, lowering his voice.

"For the time being," said Mrs. Bird, "I suggest we don't tell him anything. He'll be most upset if he thinks the whole thing is his fault."

"He really will have trouble with his 'er, ums' then," said Jonathan.

"Careful," hissed Judy, "I think he's coming downstairs. I was wondering where he'd got to."

Sure enough, a moment later the door opened

and a familiar face appeared around the gap.

"Can anyone tell me what air miles are?" asked Paddington.

"Well," said Mr. Brown, after he had gone. "That was a conversation stopper if ever I heard one. I wonder what he's up to now?"

"I shudder to think," said Mrs. Brown.

"Time alone will tell," said Mrs. Bird. "I daresay we shall know soon enough."

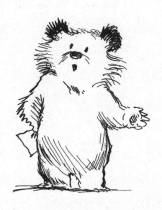

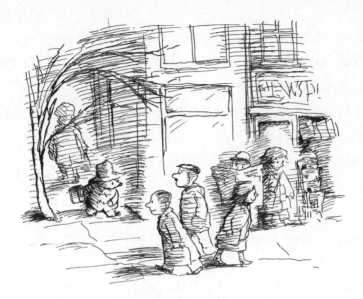

Chapter Six

PADDINGTON AIMS HIGH

THE FOLLOWING MORNING, blissfully unaware of the dark cloud that had settled over number 32 Windsor Gardens, Paddington set out soon after breakfast.

Heading in the opposite direction from the one he normally took, he made his way uphill toward a shop he remembered seeing on one of his outings with Mr. Gruber.

It was situated in a busy high street some distance from the Portobello Market, and it stuck in his mind, partly because at the time he had thought Oyster Travels seemed a very unusual name for a shop and also because there had been a large revolving globe in the window. Mr. Gruber had stopped to admire it, and as it went slowly round and round, he had pointed out all the different countries as they went past.

"Since they invented the airplane, Mr. Brown," he had said, "the world has shrunk. There are very few places left that cannot be reached in a matter of hours rather than weeks. I expect this shop took its name from the old saying: 'The world is your oyster.' In other words, 'It is yours to enjoy.'"

Mr. Gruber had a happy knack of making even quite ordinary things sound exciting, and Paddington's latest idea was far from ordinary. It had come to him during the night while he had been lying awake trying to think what to get the Browns for Christmas.

The first time he had seen the shop it had been full of people, but as he drew near he was pleased to see that apart from a rather superior-looking man who looked as though he was about to open up for business, there was nobody else around.

"The early bird catches the worm," the man said approvingly as he held the door open for Paddington.

"I daresay you'll be after one of our cheap day return trips," he said, sizing up his first customer of the day. "A day out in Brightsea perhaps? It can be very invigorating at this time of the year. The coach leaves in half an hour, and if the weather forecast is anything to go by, it will certainly blow the cobwebs out of your whiskers."

Paddington took a quick look at his reflection in the polished glass. "Those aren't cobwebs," he said, giving the man a hard stare. "It's shredded wheat. I ate my breakfast in a hurry because I wanted to get here before anyone else."

"I do beg your pardon." The man wilted under Paddington's gaze.

"I was really wanting to inquire about some of

the places you have on your globe," said Paddington. "Mr. Gruber was telling me all about them."

"My dear sir, you couldn't have come to a better place." Leaping into action, the man began washing his hands with invisible soap as he ushered Paddington to a stool opposite one of the counters.

"I happen to be the manager," he continued, going around to the other side and reaching for a pad and pencil. "As I like to tell all our customers, the world is not only our oyster, it is yours too. We are here to take care of your every need.

"Perhaps you could let me have a few details first, starting with your name and address."

Paddington did as he was bid, and while the manager was writing it down he glanced around the shop. It seemed full of interesting things. Apart from a number of real oyster shells dotted around the counter, there were some giant plastic ones hanging from the ceiling, and the walls were covered in posters showing vacationers with happy, smiling faces as they bathed in the blue sea or lay back in their deck chairs, enjoying the

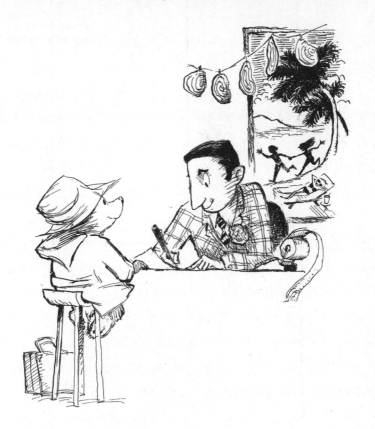

sunshine. There wasn't a gloomy face to be seen anywhere, and he felt more certain than ever that he had come to the right place.

"Will it be just for your good self?" inquired the manager. "Or will you be accompanied? We do have what we call our Singles Special."

"There will be seven of us," said Paddington. "It's

my treat, and I want to take them somewhere special for Christmas."

"Seven!" The manager took a firmer grip of his pencil. "Would you mind giving me their names?"

"Well," said Paddington, "there will be Mr. and Mrs. Brown, and Mrs. Bird. Jonathan and Judy, and I'm hoping Mr. Gruber might be able to come too."

"Quite a large party," said the manager, looking suitably impressed. Taking a closer look at Paddington, he revised his first impression. Clearly he was dealing with a seasoned traveler, and an important one at that. Although the customer had arrived on foot, he wondered for a moment if he could be dealing with a television personality planning a forthcoming program, or perhaps some kind of foreign dignitary—a slightly eccentric Indian prince down on his luck, for example. He had never met one wearing a duffle coat before, but there was a first time for everything, and one never knew these days. It paid to be careful.

"I know it's a little early in the day," he said, "but would you care for a glass of champagne while we go through the possibilities?"

"No thank you," said Paddington. "I had one once and it tickled my whiskers. I would sooner have a cup of cocoa."

The manager's face fell. "I'm afraid we shall have to wait until our Miss Pringle arrives," he said, looking at his watch. "She usually collects the milk on her way in. We were rushed off our feet yesterday," he explained, "what with everyone wanting to make a quick getaway for the Christmas holiday. I told the staff they could come in half an hour later than usual." He reached out toward a rack laden with colored brochures.

"Have you ever thought about visiting South America? The Peruvian Andes, for example? We have a tour that includes a boat trip on Lake Titicaca. As I'm sure you know, it's the highest one in the world."

"If we go to Peru," said Paddington, "I would sooner visit the Home for Retired Bears in Lima. I haven't seen my Aunt Lucy for a long time, and it will be a nice surprise for her."

The manager scanned through the brochure. "I'm afraid it doesn't mention anything about a

Home for Retired Bears," he said, "but I'm sure our tour guide will be more than willing to offer advice when you get there.

"Alternatively"—he reached for another brochure—"how would you feel about visiting India?" He held it aloft for Paddington's benefit. "Have you ever seen the Taj Mahal by moonlight?"

Paddington peered at the picture. "No," he said, "but last year I was taken to see the Christmas lights at Crumbold and Ferns."

"If I may be so bold," said the manager, "there is simply no comparison. In fact, the two can hardly be mentioned in the same breath."

"I didn't have to wait for a full moon to see Crumbold and Ferns's lights," said Paddington firmly. "They were on day and night. *And* they kept changing color. Besides, I usually go to bed early."

"If you spend more than two nights in India," said the manager, not to be outdone, "I could make sure you get a free elephant ride thrown in."

"I don't think Mrs. Bird would be very keen on that," replied Paddington. "She likes a wheel at all four corners."

"I can see I am dealing with a young gentleman of taste and discernment," said the manager, trying to mask his disappointment. "Perhaps I might tempt you with something nearer home. How about a visit to Italy and the Leaning Tower of Pisa?"

"I don't think Mrs. Bird would like that very much either," said Paddington. "She was very worried last year when Mr. Brown found a crack in the kitchen ceiling."

"Perhaps before you reach a final decision, you might care to bring the lady in?" suggested the manager. "I shall be more than happy to go through the itinerary with her."

"It's meant to be a surprise," said Paddington, "and Mrs. Bird doesn't like surprises."

"Oh, dear," said the manager through gritted teeth. "I trust she doesn't object to flying."

"When we went to France by airplane," said Paddington, "she kept her eyes closed during takeoff and landing. She said if God had meant us to fly, he would have given us wings."

"Ah," said the manager, looking slightly dazed. "I suppose the dear lady does have a point."

He tried dipping his toes in the water again. "Would Sir be thinking of traveling first or club class?"

"Whichever you think is best," said Paddington. "I want it to be a special treat."

"It depends a little on the overall cost," said the manager, trying to sum up his client.

"I'm not worried about the money," said Paddington.

"Then undoubtedly first class is best," said the manager. "I can thoroughly recommend it. It's much more restful."

"We shall need five separate rooms," said Paddington.

"They aren't exactly what you might call rooms," said the manager. "Not even on the biggest planes, unless you happen to be traveling as a guest of the United States president. But these days the seats do fold right back, and apart from the noise of the engines, once they turn the lights out you can almost believe you are in a room."

"Mrs. Bird would like that," said Paddington. "Especially if they switch the lights off."

The manager breathed a sigh of relief. "In that case," he said, washing his hands with invisible soap again, "it sounds as though our Gold Star, Top of the Range Round the World Special' would suit you down to the ground. You will be fully escorted all the way and you will stay at all the best five-star hotels, even Mrs. Bird would be hard put to find fault with the service—"

"It sounds very good value," broke in Paddington. "I think I would like one of those, please."

"In which case," said the manager, "if you intend traveling over the Christmas period, we had better strike while the iron is hot before everything gets booked up. Excuse me for a moment."

Handing Paddington some brochures to read while he was waiting, the manager turned to a nearby computer and began running his hands over the keys with practiced ease. Several minutes passed before he pressed a button, and almost immediately a long roll of paper began to emerge.

"There you are," he said, holding the end of it up for Paddington to see. "The wonders of science!

Everything you want has been confirmed. It is all down in print, including the grand total."

"Thank you very much," said Paddington as he got up to leave. "I shall always come here in the future whenever I want to go anywhere."

He reached out to take the roll of paper, but the manager kept a firm hold of the other end.

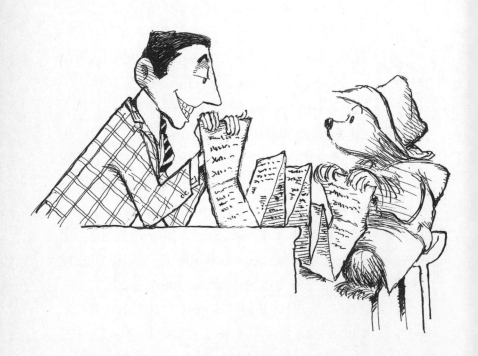

"Call me old-fashioned," he said, choosing his words with care, "and I sincerely hope you won't mind my mentioning it, but we at Oyster Travels believe in treating our customers as though they were part of one big happy family.

"To put it another way, if I may make so bold, there is the small matter of a payment in advance. You will see the total amount at the end of the form."

Paddington nearly fell off his stool as he gazed at the figure on the sheet. Far from being a small matter, it struck him as very large one. In fact, he couldn't remember ever having seen quite so many zeroes in one long line before, and he was glad he didn't have to find the money.

Reaching into his duffle coat pocket, he produced the note the man conducting the survey had given him and handed it across the counter.

The manager stared at it for several seconds, hardly able to believe his eyes. Meanwhile, the smile on his face became fixed as though it had been etched in stone.

"An air mile!" he exclaimed at last. "*One air mile!* They won't even let you on the airport bus for that! Have you not read the small print on the back?"

"I tried to," said Paddington, "but it was a bit too small, even with my magnifying glass."

Gazing heavenward, the manager placed both hands together to form a steeple. He closed his eyes, and his lips began to move as though he was very slowly counting, although no sound emerged.

After the speed at which he had operated the computer, it struck Paddington as very strange, and he wondered if the man was having trouble with all the zeroes.

"Can I help?" he asked. "Bears are good at sums."

The man's lips stopped moving, and he sat very still for a moment or two longer before opening his eyes.

"I have been counting up to ten," he explained, staring glassily at Paddington as though examining something the cat had brought in. "Having got as far as five, I am now going to close my eyes and begin again. If you are still here when I open them, I shall not be responsible for my actions. I hope I make myself clear. On your way!"

Paddington didn't wait to hear any more. Without even asking for his voucher back, he made for the door.

On his way out he bumped into a lady about to enter. Raising his hat politely, he held it open for her, and as he did he saw she was carrying several cartons of milk.

"If I were you, Miss Pringle," he said, "I wouldn't go anywhere near the man in charge. I don't think he's in a very good mood this morning."

Once he was outside, Paddington disappeared back down the hill as fast as his legs would carry him. He was vaguely aware of the sound of a car horn and someone shouting, but he didn't slow down until the green front door of number 32 Windsor Gardens had slammed shut behind him. Even then he slid one of the bolts across, just in case.

"Where *have* you been?" said Judy, as she helped him off with his duffle coat. "We've been looking for you everywhere."

While he was getting his breath back Paddington did his best to explain.

"Oh, dear," said Judy. "Poor you! But never mind. It was a lovely thought, and that's what counts the most. Besides, if we *had* gone away, you'd have missed Mrs. Bird's turkey. Who knows what we might have ended up eating instead?"

"Anyway"—she handed Paddington a half-opened package with a Peruvian stamp on it—"it's your Christmas parcel from Aunt Lucy, and I'm afraid it got stuck in the letter box."

Paddington stared at a battered Advent calendar inside the paper. It was resting on top of some table mats.

Every Christmas without fail, a parcel arrived from the Home for Retired Bears in Lima containing presents for all the family. It was one of the many ways in which the residents whiled away their time. If it wasn't jam making, it was knitting hats or weaving table mats.

Mrs. Bird would never have said anything for fear of hurting Paddington's feelings, but the mats were nothing if not long wearing, and over the years she had filled several kitchen drawers with them.

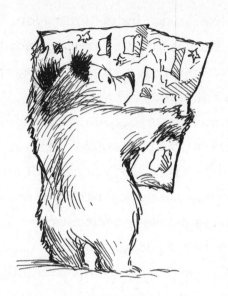

In any case, the most important item was always the calendar specially made by Aunt Lucy herself for Paddington.

"All my doors have come open!" he exclaimed hotly.

"It wasn't the postman's fault," said Judy. "For some reason there were more mats than usual, and when he tried getting it through the letter box it stuck halfway."

"Perhaps I could glue them shut," said Paddington hopefully.

"You'll never get them open again if you do," said Mrs. Bird, joining in the conversation. "Leave it with me. I'll give it a good going-over while I'm doing the ironing."

"In the meantime," said Jonathan. "No peeping."

As Mrs. Bird disappeared into the kitchen, taking the Advent calendar with her, Paddington hurried to the front door and peered through the letter box to see if by any chance the postman was still doing his rounds, but all he saw instead was a long black car driving slowly past. It was the longest one he had ever seen. In fact, it was so long he didn't think it was ever going to end, and he went back to the living room to tell Jonathan and Judy.

"It sounds like a stretch limo," said Jonathan knowedgeably.

"It was a very slow one," said Paddington. "It tried to stop, and then it went on again. I think the man driving it was looking for somewhere to park."

"I bet you couldn't see anyone in the back," said Jonathan.

Paddington shook his head. "The windows were all dark."

"That was a stretch limo all right," said Jonathan.

"It must be someone very important," said Judy.

A thought suddenly struck her. She turned to her brother. "You don't think . . . it isn't someone looking for you-know-who?"

"Who's that?" asked Paddington.

Judy put a hand to her mouth, but before she had time to answer, there was a ring at the front doorbell.

"I was right!" she cried. "What are we going to do?"

Taking hold of one of the long curtains at the French windows, Jonathan signaled to Paddington.

"Quick! Hide behind here."

Paddington had no idea what the others were talking about, but he could tell by the tones of their voices that it was urgent, and by then his knees were shaking so much he didn't wait to ask.

As soon as Paddington was safely hidden Jonathan turned back to his sister. "I told you we should have done something about making a trap-door in the floorboards for him."

Before Judy had time to answer, there was a loud sneeze.

"Pardon me!" called Paddington.

"Ssh!" said Judy.

"The curtains are tickling my nose, and I can't find my handkerchief," cried Paddington. "I think it must be in one of my duffle coat pockets."

"Too late!" groaned Jonathan, as the sound of voices drew near and the door handle began to turn.

"Guess who's here!" said Mrs. Bird.

Scanning the room, her eagle eyes immediately spotted movement behind the curtain. "You'd better come out, Paddington. There's someone to see you."

Both Jonathan and Judy stared at their visitor in amazement. Much to their relief, anything less like a government inspector would have been hard to imagine. He was much too short for a start—not a great deal taller than Paddington.

His clothes also had to be seen to be believed. Topped by a round black-brimmed hat worn squarely on his head, the bottom half, or the little of

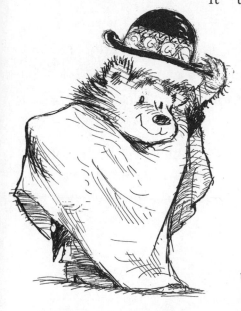

it that could be seen beneath a multi-colored cloak, was a mixture of styles. The top half appeared to be a black dinner jacket that looked as though it had seen better days, while the khaki trousers, full of bulging pockets, looked more suited to the jungle.

On the other hand, his boots were so highly polished you could have seen your face in them.

When the stranger spoke, it was with a mixture of accents, none of which they could immediately place.

"Remember me, *sobrino*?" he called. "Caught up with you at long last."

At the sound of the voice, Paddington emerged from behind the curtain and hurried across the room, paws outstretched.

"Uncle Pastuzo!" he exclaimed.

"Thank goodness for that!" whispered Judy, taking her brother's hand.

"Who would have thought it?" said Jonathan. "Wonders will never cease."

All of a sudden it felt as though the cloud that had been hanging over their heads had disappeared of its own accord.

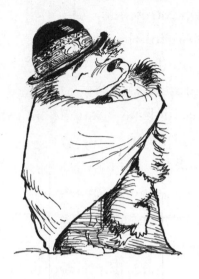

Chapter Seven

PADDINGTON'S CHRISTMAS SURPRISE

ENVELOPING PADDINGTON IN his poncho, Uncle Pastuzo gave him a huge hug. "Thought I would never find you, *sobrino*. You ask me how? Is another story. I tell you sometime.

"Been twice around the world since last July."

"You must be dying for a cup of tea," said Mrs. Brown.

Along with Mr. Brown, she had arrived on the scene rather later than the others, and they were both trying to catch up on events.

Letting go of Paddington, their visitor produced a large watch on the end of a chain. "Gone ten of the clock, and I no have breakfast yet!"

"Mercy me!" exclaimed Mrs. Bird. "I'll get you something straightaway."

Uncle Pastuzo kissed her hand. "*Gracias,* beautiful *señora,*" he said. "That is music to my ears."

"We have several kinds of cereal." Mrs. Bird went quite pink as she began ticking off various alternatives on her fingers. "There's porridge . . . kippers . . . bacon and eggs . . . sausages . . . black pudding . . . fried potato . . . toast and marmalade . . ."

"Sounds great to me, *señora!*" said Uncle Pastuzo, smacking his lips.

The Browns exchanged glances. From the back view of Mrs. Bird as she bustled off toward the kitchen it was hard to tell what she was thinking, and they feared the worst, but a moment or so later they relaxed when they heard the sound of pots and pans being put to work.

"You know something about travel?" said Uncle Pastuzo. "It makes you hungry."

"However *did* you find us?" asked Mrs. Brown.

"It was written in the stars. Heard tell on the grapevine there was a bear living in London. Had a railroad station named after him."

"I think," said Mrs. Brown gently, "you will find it was the other way around."

"That is not how it was told to me, *señora*," said Uncle Pastuzo, "so when I reach London, I head for the station, and there I see a newspaper headline. Knew at once who they were talking about."

He turned to Paddington. "Began cruising the area. Next thing I know, you are coming out of a shop that has big globe in the window."

"Oyster Travels," said Paddington.

"Right in one. So what happens? I get out of my limo and shout your name, but by then you had vanished into the crowd."

"I was hoping to take everyone around the world too," said Paddington sadly, "but I only had one air mile."

"*Sobrino*, when I get back home, you can have all mine," said Uncle Pastuzo. "By now there should be enough to take you anywhere you wish."

"I don't know anyone who's been around the world once," said Jonathan, "let alone twice."

"Took wrong path in Africa," said Uncle Pastuzo simply. "Turned right instead of left. Went back on myself. Thought everything was beginning to look the same."

"How about your car?" asked Mr. Brown. "I wouldn't want it to get towed away. They're rather hot on that kind of thing around here."

"No problem," said Uncle Pastuzo cheerfully. "Fits your front drive like a dream; all ten meters of it! Could have been made to measure."

"I'm sure Paddington's uncle will have it moved when you want to get yours out, Henry," said Mrs. Brown, catching the look on her husband's face. "Better that than have it towed away."

"Too true it is!" agreed Uncle Pastuzo. "Rules and regulations! People invent the motorcar and make things so you can't live without one. Then others come along and make it impossible to live *with* it! Poppycock!"

"Yes, well . . ." began Mr. Brown. "You try saying that to a traffic warden."

"I did," said Uncle Pastuzo. "One of them tried to give me a ticket when I came out of that oyster place. Only been in there two minutes."

Producing a giant dagger from under his poncho, he ran his free paw along the length of the blade. "I tell him, 'You want to watch it, *gringo!*'"

"Oh, dear," said Mrs. Brown. "I hope you didn't give him our address."

Uncle Pastuzo chuckled. "Me? I was not born yesterday. Gave him your neighbor's number. *Hombre* name of Curry. Heard all about him from Lucy. Seems you two don't get on too well."

"You are in touch with Paddington's Aunt Lucy?" said Mrs. Brown, anxious to change the subject.

"First stop when I set out," said Uncle Pastuzo. "There she was, large as life and twice as happy in the Home for Retired Bears. Knitting away in her rocking chair like there was no tomorrow. Could hardly hear myself think for all the needles clicking: tea cozies, bed socks, scarves . . . you call that retirement?

"She tell me your address. Only thing is, I remember the number of your house but forget the name of the road. Not like Darkest Peru. Where I live we only got one. Straight up to the top of the mountain and straight back down again. Got the rest of the address from that oyster place. That was when I know it was meant."

He turned to Paddington. "Spoke to man in there with bad twitch. Said he knew you well, *sobrino*. Seems like you are not the apple of his eye."

"You will be staying, of course," broke in Mrs. Brown. "We can make a room ready while you are having your breakfast."

Uncle Pastuzo glanced out at the garden. "No need," he said, pointing to the summer house. "Give me hammer and nail, and that will suit me just fine. Like a palace."

"Are you sure?" asked Mrs. Brown. "Won't you be cold?"

"You haven't slept outside in the Andes in the middle of winter," said Uncle Pastuzo.

"That's true," admitted Mrs. Brown.

"Wake up most mornings with icicles on your whiskers. Those that have them," he added hastily, not wishing to offend.

"I'd better move the lawn mower," said Mr. Brown.

He paused. "Er . . . forgive my asking, but why do you need a hammer and a nail?"

"Need somewhere to hang this." Uncle Pastuzo reached for his hat. "Home is where you hang it."

With a quick flick he sent his hat flying across the room. It hovered for a brief moment near the ceiling before landing gently on top of a standard lamp.

"Gosh!" said Jonathan admiringly. "I wish I could do that."

"I teach you," said Uncle Pastuzo. "Is what they call a knack."

"It may be a knack," said Mrs. Brown, fearing for her china, "but it might not be so easy with a school cap."

"Meantime," said Uncle Pastuzo, ignoring the interruption, "I give *Señora* Bird a hand. Make sure she does eggs the way I like. Over easy, sunny-side up."

"May I come too?" asked Paddington eagerly.

The Browns looked at each other when they were on their own.

"What do you think he meant when he said home is where you hang your hat?" asked Mrs. Brown. "It sounded a bit permanent to me."

"How long is a piece of string?" said Mr. Brown. "I know one thing; if breakfast is anything to go by, we'd better get some more supplies in before the shops close for Christmas."

In the end it was Mrs. Bird who answered most of their questions. Clearly she couldn't wait to unburden herself when she returned at long last.

"That should keep them quiet for a while," she said, undoing her apron. "Besides, there is a lot of catching up to do. I've left Paddington in charge of the toast and marmalade."

"Tell us the worst," said Mr. Brown.

"Well . . ."—Mrs. Bird took a deep breath—"Paddington's uncle lives high up in the Andes mountains in an area that is rich in all kinds of precious metals: copper, gold, silver . . . platinum. Now, who do you think benefits the most?"

"The people who dig for it?" suggested Jonathan.

"Wrong," said Mrs. Bird.

"Their employers?" hazarded Judy.

"Wrong again," said Mrs. Bird.

"If the car parked in our front drive is anything to go by," said Mr. Brown, "Uncle Pastuzo."

"Right," said Mrs. Bird. "He has a little store at the top of one of the biggest mines, and when the workers come up at the end of their shift, hot, tired, and above all thirsty, he's there ready and waiting with hot dogs and ice-cold drinks.

"They may have spent their time underground looking for precious metals, but Uncle Pastuzo has his own gold mine at the top. In any case, there is nowhere else to spend their earnings.

"Having grown wealthy over the years, he now wants to see a bit of the world while he can. As he says, you can't take it with you."

"He told you all that while you were cooking his breakfast?" said Mrs. Brown.

"And a lot more besides," said Mrs. Bird. "There's nothing like getting together over a kitchen stove to make people open up."

"Er . . . while you were chatting, did you get any idea of how long he plans to stay?" asked Mr. Brown.

"As far as I'm concerned," said Mrs. Bird, "he can make it as long as he likes.

"He has the same big brown eyes as certain others I could name," she added dreamily, "and he's very polite. You can see where Paddington gets it from—along with his Aunt Lucy, of course."

"So what more can you tell us?" asked Mrs. Brown.

"Just you wait and see," said Mrs. Bird mysteriously. "It's his idea and I wouldn't want to spoil it, especially as it's meant to be a surprise for Paddington."

And there, for the time being, matters rested.

After his mammoth breakfast, Paddington's uncle

went outside to his car and returned carrying a suitcase. Laying it down in the middle of the floor, he opened the lid and pressed a button, and a small folding bed began to erect itself. It was followed by a whirr and a hiss of air as a mattress took shape.

"Bought it in Hong Kong," he said briefly.

"Are you sure you wouldn't like something bigger?" asked Mrs. Brown.

Uncle Pastuzo shook his head. "They say that to me when I stay at the Ritz hotel in Paris, France. They no like it when I say I prefer my bed to theirs. I tell them, if they no let me use my bed, then I camp out in front of their hotel and hang my washing out to dry. They like that even less."

"It's a wonder they didn't have you arrested," said Mr. Brown.

Uncle Pastuzo jingled some coins in a trouser pocket. "Not so as you would notice . . . *buenas noches.*"

Having said good night, Paddington's uncle opened the French windows, gathered his belongings together, and headed toward the summer house.

"I'd better move the lawn mower," said Mr. Brown.

"Don't forget the hammer and nails," called Mrs. Brown.

"It must be nice to be so independent," she continued, closing the door after them. "But it is rather unsettling for the rest of us. I wonder when he wants to be woken?"

"I should leave him be for the time being," said Mrs. Bird. "It's best to let sleeping bears lie."

"Perhaps he's hibernating," suggested Jonathan.

"Our geography mistress says bears don't hibernate in the true sense of the word," said Judy. "On the other hand, some of them do go to sleep for months at a time. Perhaps we should ask Paddington?"

"Don't put ideas into that bear's head," warned Mrs. Bird. "He has more than enough in there already."

As things turned out, however, they were all wrong about Uncle Pastuzo. The next morning he was up bright and early, and after announcing he "had matters to deal with," disappeared soon after breakfast and didn't arrive back until late that afternoon.

"If you don't mind my asking," said Mrs. Brown, "what do you picture doing for the rest of the day?"

"You mean, what are *we* doing?" said Uncle Pastuzo.

There was a toot from the limousine outside.

"Better hurry," said Uncle Pastuzo. "Otherwise we miss flight."

"Miss the flight?" echoed the Browns.

"That is what they call it," said Uncle Pastuzo, ushering everyone out of the door.

Climbing into the front seat, he settled down alongside the driver and began issuing instructions. But they were lost on the Browns as they entered via the rear doors.

Paddington nearly fell over backward with surprise when he climbed inside. The last person he expected to see was Mr. Gruber, seated in an armchair at the far end.

"It is a small world, Mr. Brown," said his friend. "And as I think I once said to you, it gets smaller all the time. I feel very honored to have been invited."

"It's very James Bond," said Judy, eyeing a bank of television screens.

"Everything except a nuclear warhead," agreed Jonathan.

"I don't think I could live with those curtains," said Mrs. Bird, casting an expert eye over the furnishings. "They're far too grand, and they don't go with the carpet."

"I hope we don't come across anyone we know," said Mrs. Brown, settling herself down in another armchair. "Perhaps we'd better draw them just in case."

"They won't be able to see us," said Jonathan, pointing to the tinted glass, "but if you like . . ." Running his eyes over a control console in front of them, he pressed a button and the curtains slid together.

"Do *you* know what's happening, Mr. Gruber?" asked Paddington.

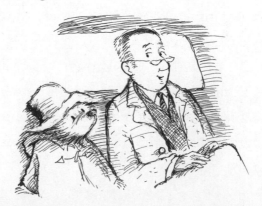

But Mr. Gruber wasn't letting on. "It is something I have always wanted to do, Mr. Brown" was all he would say.

Mrs. Bird was equally tight-lipped on the subject, and for most of the journey everyone else was kept so busy trying out the various gadgets they hardly noticed where they were going anyway.

When they eventually drew to a halt Jonathan pressed the button again, and as the curtains parted he and Judy joined Paddington at one of the windows.

"Guess what!" said Jonathan.

"It looks like a bicycle wheel to me," said Paddington.

"It's called the London Eye," said Judy.

"We're all going for a ride on it," explained Mr. Gruber.

"We're going for a ride on a bicycle wheel!" exclaimed Paddington. "I hope we don't get a puncture!"

"There's no fear of that," said Mr. Gruber. "If you take a closer look, you will see there are lots of cabins all around the rim. We shall be traveling in one of those."

"They look as though they are made of glass," said Judy. "They aren't, of course, but it does mean you can look every which way while you are going around."

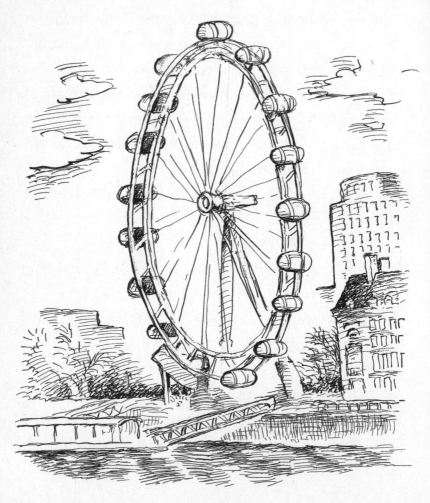

"And you can stand up and walk around," added Jonathan.

"Thirty-two of them," said Uncle Pastuzo, helping the others disembark from the car. "Each one holds twenty-five passengers. That is nearly eight hundred people. I book through your friend at the oyster shop, *sobrino*, and I pay extra so we have a whole one to ourselves. He is so pleased he say any time you want a holiday you go see him."

"Mrs. Bird's right," whispered Jonathan. "Bears *do* fall on their feet."

"I fix everything," said Uncle Pastuzo, as a hostess came forward to greet them. "We take what is called the VIP trip. Tee hee!"

"Tee hee?" repeated Mrs. Brown.

"Ought to be VIB—Very Important Bears!"

Doubled up with laughter at his own joke, Uncle Pastuzo followed on behind their escort.

The timing was exactly right. As they arrived at the starting point, an empty capsule arrived. The doors slid open, and as they stepped aboard, the sun began to disappear behind the Houses of Parliament.

For the first few minutes, as the wheel slowly

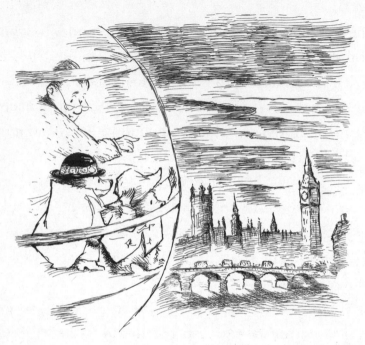

revolved and they gathered height, Mr. Gruber
pointed out many of the important landmarks still
visible in the gathering dusk to Paddington's uncle:
Big Ben; Buckingham Palace; the Tower of
London; St. Paul's cathedral; the many parks and
lakes; and the British Telecom Tower, silhouetted
like a pencil against the skyline.

Paddington had visited many of them over the
years, but somehow, as London began to unfold
before his eyes, they seemed to take on a different life,

the buildings evolving into tiny scale models of the real thing, the streets peopled by ants and model cars going hither and thither everywhere he looked.

"Is the only way to see the world," said Uncle Pastuzo, pleased at everyone's reaction. "From on high and away from the crowds."

As darkness fell still further and the capsule gradually rose higher and higher, lights began appearing all over London. Floodlit buildings came into view, and Christmas lights twinkled in the night sky.

They even had a brief glimpse of ice-skaters on the far side of the river farther around to their right.

There was one slight hiccup almost at the end of its journey, when Uncle Pastuzo called them all together to see what he called "something special," but by the time they had formed themselves into a group, the moment had passed.

It had been one long series of magical moments, and in the rush to disembark, nobody noticed Uncle Pastsuzo disappear for a minute or two. In any case they had grown used to his sudden comings and goings.

On the journey home Paddington joined in the general agreement that it was the best treat they'd had for a very long time.

All the same, Mrs. Bird couldn't help noticing that in between whiles both Paddington and his uncle were unusually quiet.

She couldn't help wondering if all the talk about going around the world and now the trip on the London Eye had given Paddington itchy paws, but for the time being she kept her thoughts to herself. There was no sense in spoiling everyone else's pleasure.

Uncle Pastuzo dropped Mr. Gruber off first.

"You have been a good friend over the years to my *sobrino*," he said, shaking him warmly by the hand. "For that I bless you."

Somehow as Mr. Gruber waved good-bye, it all seemed very final.

The Browns' housekeeper had difficulty in getting to sleep that night, and the result was she woke rather later than usual the next morning. Even so, the house felt strangely quiet.

Slipping into a dressing gown, she was making her way downstairs when she happened to glance out of the landing window and realized Uncle Pastuzo's car was no longer in the driveway.

Her heart missing a beat, she hastened back upstairs to Paddington's room. The duvet was pulled back and there was a hollow in the mattress where he must have lain, but it felt cold to the touch.

On the way down again she found two envelopes lying on the front door mat. The one marked "*Señora Bird*" she put into her apron pocket for later; the other was marked for Mr. and Mrs. Brown.

Soon the whole household was awake to her calls, and everyone came rushing downstairs to see what the excitement was about.

The note to Mr. and Mrs Brown was typically short.

"Been there, done that, now is time to go home," read Mr. Brown. "So, *amigos*, it is time to say *adiós* and *gracias*."

"That's nice," he said, once he had got over the initial shock. "Somehow *adiós* sounds better than good-bye; it's not quite so final."

"And *gracias* is so much better than a simple 'thank you,'" agreed Mrs. Brown.

"The thing is," said Mrs. Bird, searching for the right words and hardly able to find the right ones to say what was uppermost in her mind. "Where's Paddington?"

Something in the tone of her voice caused a ripple of apprehension to run through the others.

"He was out in the garden the last time I saw him," said Jonathan. "I think he was doing some early-morning digging."

One glance through the dining-room window was enough.

Paddington nearly dropped his seaside spade with surprise when he suddenly found himself surrounded by the rest of the family.

"I was looking for some buried treasure," he

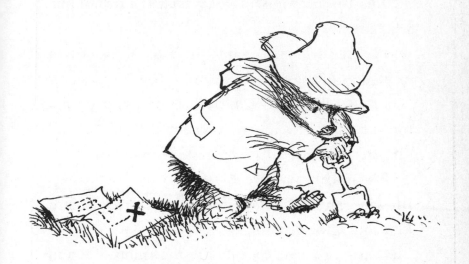

announced. "Uncle Pastuzo left me a map he made.

"He doesn't like good-byes, so he slipped it under my door last night after I went to bed." He held it up for the others to see. "I thought I'd better get up early in case Mr. Curry saw me and wanted to know what I was doing."

"X marks the spot where you start," said Jonathan, looking at the roughly drawn map.

"It says ten paces north," said Judy. "Then five paces east."

"The trouble is," said Paddington, "I'm not sure which is north."

"I'll get my spade," said Mr. Brown, by now as excited as the rest of them.

Having followed the instructions, he ended up in the shrubbery. That's my prize buddleia," he said. "It can't be under that. At least, I hope it isn't."

"It's probably a case of bear's paces," said Mrs. Brown. "They're not as long as ours. You'd better let Paddington have a go."

Having first been pointed in the right direction, Paddington set out while the others counted the steps as he went.

Sure enough, this time the trail ended in the middle of a flower bed. Mr. Brown brushed aside a pile of leaves to reveal a freshly dug patch of earth, and after a few prods with his spade he struck metal.

"Brilliant!" exclaimed Jonathan.

"I don't know about that," said Mr. Brown. "It's the box I keep my golf balls in. I hope they're all right."

"Do hurry up, Henry," called Mrs. Brown. "Paddington's waiting."

"Why don't you have a go then," said Mr. Brown, handing him the spade.

Paddington needed no second bidding, and in no time at all he prized the box out of the ground and had the lid open.

The first thing he came across was a canvas bag with his name on the tag. Pulling on the drawstrings, he felt inside and discovered it was full of foreign coins.

"Uncle Pastuzo must have collected them while he was traveling around the world," said Jonathan, taking a closer look. "I bet they're worth a fortune!"

Underneath that, carefully wrapped in tissue paper, were seven large glossy photographs of the whole family taken inside the capsule on the London Eye.

"So that's where he disappeared to," said Judy. "I saw a notice on the way in saying if you pose at a certain point a picture is automatically taken, ready to buy when you get off."

"What a very kind thought," said Mrs. Brown. "We must have ours framed, Henry. It can have a

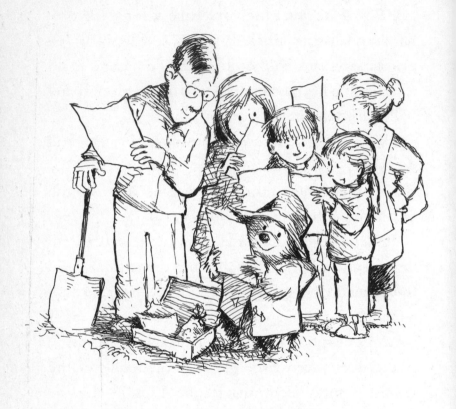

place of honor on the mantelpiece."

"I shall put mine by my bed," said Mrs. Bird.

"We can take ours with us when we go back to school," added Judy.

"And I shall put mine alongside Aunt Lucy's picture," said Paddington. "I'll give Mr. Gruber his tomorrow. I expect he would like it for the shop."

"We shall miss Uncle Pastuzo," said Mrs. Brown on the way back to the house.

"He may have been a bit of a whirlwind, but it will seem very quiet without him."

"At least that bear's ends are tied up now," said Mrs. Bird. "It's always bothered me."

Having overheard the conversation, as soon as he got indoors Paddington hurried upstairs to his bedroom and examined his reflection carefully in the mirror.

As ever, Mrs. Bird was right. He had no idea how or when it had happened, but Uncle Pastuzo must have done a good job. Everything was in its proper place. No matter which way he turned, he couldn't see the slightest sign of any knots.

Later on that morning the Browns heard the sound of hammering coming from Paddington's room, but everyone was so pleased by the fact that he was still with them, they pretended not to notice.

"I've been following Aunt Lucy's example," he

announced that evening when they all went up to his room to say good night. "I've been counting my blessings. Except, I wanted to do mine *before* I go to sleep. I have so many I may not have time tomorrow.

"I still have some important shopping to do and I shall need to go to the bank to get all Uncle Pastuzo's coins counted."

"I don't think you will be very popular with the rest of the queue at this time of the year," warned Mr. Brown.

"Anyway," said Mrs. Brown, "you mustn't go spending the money on us. Your being here is the best present we could possibly have."

"Life just wouldn't be the same without you," added Mrs. Bird amid general agreement.

Paddington pointed to a large nail on the back of his bedroom door. "Uncle Pastuzo taught me one thing," he explained. "Home is where you hang your hat."

Removing his bush hat, he tossed it in the air. Much to his surprise, it landed back on his head.

"Never mind, Paddington," said Mrs. Brown amid the laughter that followed. "Practice makes perfect, and from now on you have all the time in the world!"

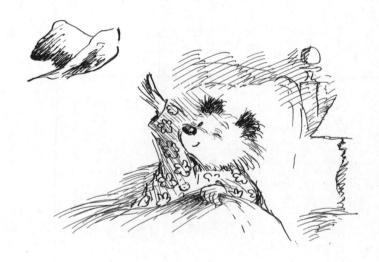

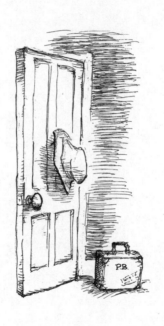